All **You** Should **Know** About

Digestive System and Liver Ailments

All **You** Should **Know** About

Digestive System and Liver Ailments

S.N. KHOSLA

PEACOCK BOOKS

An Imprint of Atlantic Publishers & Distributors

Published by
PEACOCK BOOKS
B-2, Vishal Enclave, New Delhi-110 027
Phones : 2541 3460, 2542 9987, 2546 6842

Distributed by
ATLANTIC PUBLISHERS AND DISTRIBUTORS
7/22, Ansari Road, Darya Ganj, New Delhi-110 002
Phones : 2327 3880, 2327 5880, 2328 0451
Fax : 91-11-2328 5873
E-mail : info@atlanticbooks.com
Web : www.atlanticbooks.com

Peacock Books is an imprint of
Atlantic Publishers and Distributors

Printed in India at Nice Printing Press, Delhi

To the Memory of
My Parents

PREFACE

Diseases of the abdomen and liver are of common occurence and continue to remain a challenge all over the world, more so in tropical countries.

A lot of myths are associated with some of the common abdominal ailments like gas formation, heartburn and constipation etc. A great majority of people in our country suffer from these disorders. More than 90 per cent of the Indian population suffers from amoebiasis. Abdominal ailments are often associated with poor personal hygiene, unhealthy environment and impure water supply.

The same holds true for liver diseases like hepatitis. Moreover, a poor understanding of ills of alcohol abuse often leads to liver damage.

Medicine is fast changing and also the spectrum of various diseases. The basic principles of health and hygiene, however, will remain the same.

It is our endeavor, in this book, to educate the lay people about the common diseases affecting the abdomen and the liver so that, by understanding the disease and its ill effects, preventive measures can be adopted and health care does not suffer.

S.N. Khosla

CONTENTS

INTRODUCTION

Liver is a large and a complex organ of the body and performs a number of functions — some simple, some complex.

It has got such diverse functions which range from utilising for the body the food we consume and then acting as a storehouse of energy but at the same time eliminating toxic substances it cannot take.

It performs the functions of a bodyguard fighting the evil forces inside the body with great elan. Its capacity for regeneration is unique. It has great capacity to withstand insults to the body.

Liver being such a vital organ is surprisingly least understood and less talked about by the lay fraternity. Every few years an epidemic of hepatitis brought on by floods, inadequate water supply or defective sewage disposal occurs somewhere in the country and then people become aware of what they call 'yellow peril'.

It is surprising that so little is said and being written about this vital organ. What is required is an understanding about the role of liver in our day-to-day lives and the numerous ailments being brought about by it. Following few elementary principles of basic and preventive medical care may go a long way in preventing and protecting from the morbidity and mortality of diseases associated with disturbed liver functions.

Role of alcohol vis-à-vis cirrhosis is often disputed. Cirrhosis is now one of the leading killers in modern-day lists of killer diseases, but interestingly, though its onslaught can be halted to some extent, yet very little attention is being paid to it. Liver responds to various toxins in a peculiar way and often this reaction is unpredictable.

This monograph has been written with the purpose of bringing attention to some common ailments of liver which should be given as much importance by the lay people as is being given to cardiac or other related ailments. A little understanding shall go a long way in the prevention of such ailments.

Liver demands respect from us. Let us conclude in the words of famous poet Pablo Neurda who in his poem 'Ode to the Liver' says:

Dark Monarch
Giver of syrups and poisons
regulator of salts/from you I hope
for justice
I love life. Do not betray me!
work on!
Do not arrest my song

Let us say 'Amen' to this beautiful poem and pray for a healthy liver and a Robust and kicking life.

1
YOU AND YOUR LIVER

Lying in the upper part of abdomen on the right side, liver is a master organ which controls the orchestra of the body metabolism of various important and vital energy giving substances like proteins, fats and carbohydrates.

It is also body's largest organ weighing about 1200-1500 g and comprises one-fiftieth of the total body weight. In infants and children the brain is larger than the liver but as the child grows the liver also grows along with the result that by the time the child grows up to its adulthood, the liver will have taken up the first place in size.

It is a vital organ without which life cannot be sustained for long periods and in fact for not more than 36 hours. Surprisingly liver has enormous capacity for regeneration, a property which is not shared by any other organ in the body. You cut away parts of other organs and the loss is permanent. But when a part of liver is removed it regenerates with newly grown tissue quickly and that is why the thread of life can be maintained with a very small viable liver tissue. One is familiar with the well-known Greek mythological tale where Prometheus was chained to a rock to the lonely peak of a mountain and to ensure an everlasting torture, ZEUS, the king of heaven and hearth ordered that a vulture should each day devour the Titan Prometheus liver. Each night the liver would regenerate for next day food for the vulture to feed upon, thus illustrating the immortality of liver and its regenerating capacity.

To look at, sheltered by the bony cage of the chest on the right side, the liver looks like a pyramid and its upper border almost lies approximately at the level of the nipples. Liver is mainly divided into two lobes, the right and the left. The right lobe is bigger one, and is almost six times the size of the left lobe.

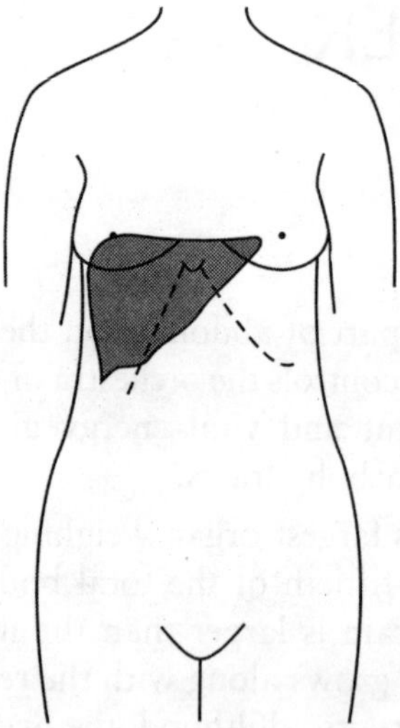

Position of Liver in Body

Liver is a very vascular organ and may hold up to four pints of blood, depending on as to how much blood is needed in other parts of the body.

It has got dual blood supply, one source is venous blood being brought by the portal veins from the intestines and spleen while the arterial blood is supplied by the hepatic artery. These vessels enter the organ through a fissure, called porta hepatis and divide to form branches which go to the various parts of the organ. All the impure or venous blood pass out through the hepatic veins which come out of the back of the liver and enter into the big channel called the inferior vena cava which ultimately enters right side of the heart.

A heavy and a large organ it is kept in position by ligaments and by means of abdominal pressure which is transmitted by the abdominal wall muscles tone. Any disease which occurs on the right side of chest or abdomen displaces the liver either up or down, depending upon where the disease is.

In some people, the liver gets displaced downwards and its anchorage becomes loose either because of a flabby abdomen or loss of elasticity of the abdominal muscles and the liver may become palpable lower down. This condition may not require much treatment and is considered normal.

Normally liver is not palpable in the abdomen except the left lobe especially in infants. But when liver is palpable in the abdomen, it indicates that there may be disease like hepatitis, heart failure, cancer, etc. Diseases of the lungs like Emphysema or Pleural Effusion may displace the liver down. It is said that some athletes or singers may by practice be experts in pushing the liver down. So if you have one of such people where otherwise there is no disease but the liver is palpable, this may be considered normal and ignored.

As said earlier, liver like an orchestra carries out a number of assorted tasks vital to the body's functioning and keeps the body in fit position. That is why when people feel out of sorts they say that they have got a 'liverish' feeling.

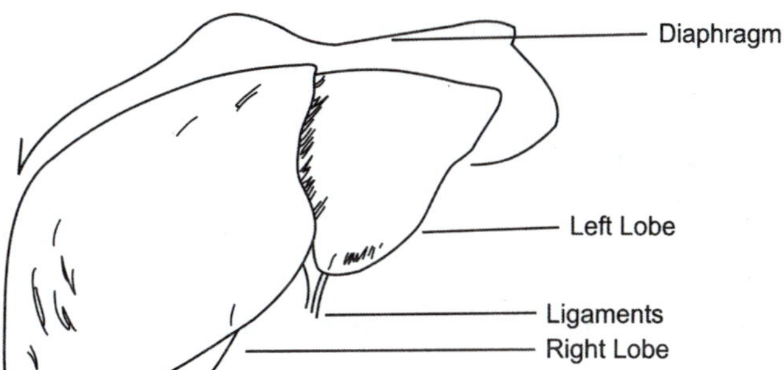

Liver: As it Looks

Basically, liver is a biochemical workshop which releases numerous essential substances into the blood and digestive system, enabling the body to get maximum benefit from the food. These are the substances which are essentially playing a major role in sustaining it because without these we cannot live.

Liver has important role to play in carbohydrate metabolism. One of the vital energy reserves of the body is a carbohydrate called glycogen or animal starch. Liver acts as a storehouse of glycogen which can be stored in large amounts in it. At times of stress, glucose is released from glycogen stores of the liver into the body. In states of starvation, body's sugar levels are maintained at normal levels for approximately twenty four hours drawing upon their reserves in the liver. Similarly proteins are synthesized in the liver and also stored to some extent. Liver produces 150-250g of proteins daily. It is the sole source of albumin 13-20g being made daily. These levels are severely effected in diseases of liver like cirrhosis. It also acts as a great storehouse of fat soluble vitamins A and D. One reason why one can go on without any appreciable ill effects of vitamin A deficiency is that as long as the liver has played its role in laying down a good supply of this vitamin beforehand, there is not going to be much difficulty. Fish liver is a good source of not only vitamin A but also of vitamin D. Normally liver contains about 5 per cent of fat by weight but excessive accumulation may take place in people taking excessive amount of alcohol or those suffering from protein-calorie malnutrition. Accumulation of fat in excess amounts ranging up to 50 per cent of the body weight is not desirable and means number of ill effects on the normal body functions. Dietary fat is transported to the liver in simpler forms like triglycerides or fatty acids. Fatty acids are converted to phospholipids and cholesterol which are excreted in the bile.

Cholesterol is also mainly synthesized by the liver and its rate of production is controlled by the amount of fat taken in the diet and by its absorption in the intestines.

An important role of liver is the storage of elements like zinc, copper and iron which are essential in the making of red corpuscles as well as improving the body's haemoglobin. Thus liver acts as a central location for the synthesis of number of substances and at the same time controlling their formation and utilization.

The liver cells form and secrete bile which is stored in the gall bladder and discharged into the intestinal tract. Bile makes possible the digestion of fats by acting as a powerful emulsifying agent. Fats in the food are broken into small droplets and then digested by the intestinal juices. This absence of bile in the intestines results in non-absorption of fats from the food and the person suffers from fatty dyspepsia and diarrhoea.

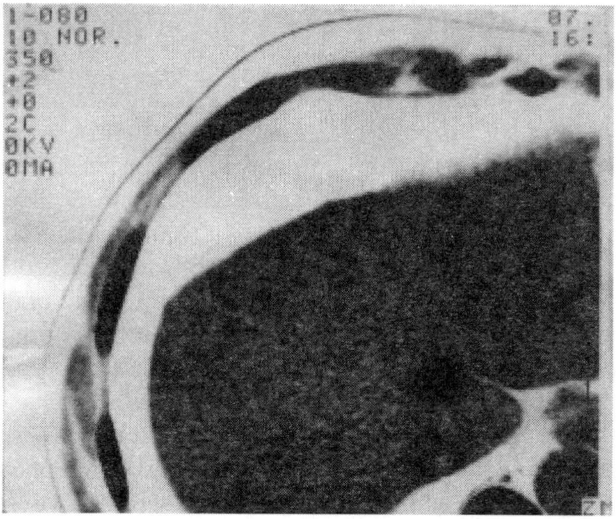

CT Scan showing magnified view of normal liver

Red blood cells in the body have a limited life and are constantly being destroyed and replaced by newer ones. The red colouring material derived from these cells is being collected by the liver and channelized into the bile. At least 75 per cent of the bilirubin produced daily is being got from broken down cells and metabolized in the liver.

Normally bilirubin is broken down by bacteria in the intestines to urobilinogen. Of this 10 to 20 per cent is reabsorbed and taken up by the liver cells. It is re-excreted into the bile but some of it passes into the general circulation and is excreted in the urine.

Any process which interferes with the normal manufacture, synthesis, utilization or excretion of bilirubin in the body is going to produce excessive accumulation of bilirubin in the body, thus giving a yellowish colouring to the skin and body tissues.

A very important role of liver is in the control of blood-clotting mechanism since liver dysfunction is going to produce bleeding from various sources. It is a complex cycle but the role of liver can be simplified when we say that liver synthesizes prothrombin which plays an important role in clotting of blood. Besides this liver plays an important link in blood-clotting mechanism and if this gets deranged it may be difficult to control bleeding from sites small or large.

If liver is storehouse of vital body foods and vitamins then it also acts as a sort of policeman guarding the human body from the ill effects of many harmful organisms and bacteria. Liver not only captures bacteria but also detoxifies substances like drugs and hormones. Inactivation of toxic substances maintains the body's equitable fight against all the trash being ingested by the body. Thus when liver fails, the body is going to fall under the deleterious effects of these drugs or hormones. Every organ has its capacity. Some food stuffs like Jamaican bush tea, senecio (a plant growing in the wheat fields of South Africa and harvested with the grain) alfotoxin (produced by certain molds growing on peanuts and cereals), etc. are substances which damage the liver. The liver can fight these dangerous substances up to certain levels but excessive and regular use is going to overpower the liver's resistance and ultimately results in liver damage.

Liver has great ability to withstand insults being inflicted on it both from inside and outside the body. To fight these, factors inside and outside the body which are interlinked come into play. The integrity of liver shall depend on adequate blood supply (to the liver and to the other parts of the body), maintenance of blood pressure in the body at normal levels. constant oxygen supply and keeping the temperature at viable levels. At the same time nutrients in adequate proportions must be supplied to keep the lifeline going.

The extent to which these alterations in any of the above conditions causes bodily dysfunction of the liver will vary from person to person as well as other innumerable factors which are regulating the functioning of the liver.

Age and sex have an important role to play in maintaining a healthy liver. Liver in very young children and old or debilitated persons is at a higher level of risk proneness. Some people have either a genetic or individual sensitivity to certain drugs. Female hormones in excess in the body may predispose to liver injury. Environmental factors have also an important bearing on the health of liver. In this group shall be included, nutrition and drugs which may have a cause and effect relationship.

Further health of liver shall be controlled by the fact whether any damage done to liver is shortlived, reversible or not. An irreversible and progressive injury to liver means failure of liver to fight.

Thus one would appreciate that liver acts like a highly organized system and has multifaceted roles to play which range from metabolism of important substances, secretion and excretion as well as detoxification of harmful substances to storage of carbohydrates, fats, proteins, etc. No wonder it is a life-saving organ which controls the well-being of the body.

LIVER AND DIET

2

Nutrition has an important role to play in the smooth functioning of body's vital functions and protecting it from its external as well as internal enemies. This is achieved partly in raising the body's defence mechanism. All important organs of the body have significant contribution to make in this regard but liver is one organ whose role is important in this regard. Other systems may stand up to any deficiency in the diet and so does the liver but often the main strain of it may fall upon this organ. There are no two opinions that diet can contribute to the disorders of the liver and the complexities of nutrition vis-à-vis liver may make its assessment often difficult.

A normal human diet is constituted by carbohydrates, proteins, fats, vitamins and minerals. What is essential and is oft stressed is the importance of a balanced nutritious diet which should be able to sustain the individual's caloric needs, depending on his/her age, occupation, physical habits and economic status. Liver acts as a storehouse of almost all the essential ingredients of the food and is often called upon to meet the body's needs at times of stress and strain.

What is really an ideal diet which not only is nutritious, energy-giving but also protective for the liver has to be considered best suited for an individual. When we talk of a diet and its role in the body's normal functioning vis-à-vis liver we should try to look at a well balanced nutritious diet which can supply the body its basic nutrients and vitamins.

A balanced diet is one which is appetizing and contains all the essential nutrients. A diet of this type need not be so simple that it does not evoke any appetite in the person and appears to be monotonous. Similarly, palate-tickling foods and richly made dishes also do not constitute the ideal diet for liver, since all these diets containing rich gravies and fats are going to take inordinate delay to digest and there is also the very significant danger that these people are going to have indigestion and essentially a sluggish liver.

Nutrition in any individual must be adequate, as malnutrition is going to act as a contributing factor in the causation as well as evolution of liver diseases. Common example in this regard is cirrhosis of liver. There is no doubt that malnutrition per se does not give rise to cirrhosis but there is much circumstantial evidence which shows that this is one major factor contributing towards it. The role of liver is quite apparent when one considers that food after digestion is absorbed from the intestines and passed into the portal vessels and then carried to the liver. Thus any poisonous or noxious substance present in the diet is going to be transported first to the liver which shall act rather as a guard for the body. It should be apparent from the above that whatever we eat must first show its credentials to the liver.

Proteins are essential for the body tissues repair which are constantly subjected to wear and replacement. Though dietary proteins are also source of energy but in this respect they are less important than the carbohydrates (starches) or fats. The protein content of the body may not be constant but depends to some extent on the proteins in the diet. There is no doubt that adequate quantities of proteins are required essentially in the diet. Most human diets provide from 10 to 15 per cent of the energy in the form of proteins. The nutritive value of the proteins shall depend to an important extent on the relationship of the aminoacids in its molecule to those required for the repair and building of new tissues. Animal foods are good source of first class proteins but it does not mean that good class of proteins cannot be derived from vegetable sources. Thus one finds that rich source of good quality proteins shall be groundnuts, milk, beans, peas, soya bean, fish, meat and eggs. Adequate quantities of proteins can be derived from wheat, rice, potatoes, millet and beans etc.

What is required in diet is mixture of both animal and vegetable proteins, since deficiency in the quality of one sort of protein shall be made good by the other protein constituents of the food.

If the intake or supply of proteins in the diet is inadequate, the body cells shall be deprived of important aminoacids for their synthetic activities. The effect is that there is overall slowing down of growth. Protein synthesis and storage is interfered with. There is failure of the liver to maintain its normal functioning and structure. There is excessive accumulation of fat in the liver and we get what is called a fatty liver. This has been shown not only in human beings but also by animal experiments. Diets low in proteins when fed to rats have resulted in the production of fatty changes in the liver. Surprisingly these changes developed in rats only if the diets were also low in vitamin E. Similarly in humans, diet low in proteins makes the liver not only fatty but also more susceptible to effects of chemical poisons and toxins. Fatty infiltration of the liver, if allowed to progress, will result in necrosis of the liver cells. In experiments on rats it has also been observed that animals fed on protein-deficient diets developed acute necrosis of the liver which ultimately resulted in death of the animal.

What is seen in experimental animals can also be seen in humans. When one talks about protein deficiency and its role in protective mechanism for the liver, one must not ignore the fact that deficiency of proteins may be produced in many ways, i.e. either the intake is poor because of economic reason, the quality of proteins are poor because of bad eating habits, religious and social taboos or the proteins in diet are being sidetracked by the regular and continued use of alcohol. Statistics from all over the world show that in poor countries and in developed countries at periods of stress like war and famine, the incidence of protein malnutrition increases manifold and with it goes up the incidence of liver cirrhosis in the general population. While poor nations suffer from lack of adequate and good nutrition for its people, the richer and affluent nations reel under the effect of alcoholism which is a major factor responsible for damaging the liver.

The incidence of liver damage vis-à-vis poor protein intake coupled with alcoholism is on the increase in Europe, America and England. Though diet plays an important role in it, yet it is not the only one to be blamed. There are other factors like food-poisoning, drugs and infections which also play a role in furthering liver damage.

The fact that liver cirrhosis is produced to large extent by deficiency of dietary protein has led to studies which have indicated that defective diets in alcoholics are because of their spending more money on alcohol and then taking poor diets. At the same time those alcoholics who continue taking good nourishing diet suffer less from serious liver disease and to some extent whatever damage occurs in the liver can be reversed up to certain level.

If the factor of adequate nutrition and proteins is essential for protecting the liver, it is equally important that quality of food should also be improved. The point in question is brought home well by the example of Indian childhood cirrhosis. Though number of factors are considered to be responsible for the causation of this disease yet some interesting observations are worth mentioning. This disease generally involves Hindu children in Bengal and amongst the Brahmin community in the South. Though Mohammedan children are also effected, yet it is very uncommon among European or Anglo-Indian children. From Punjab, the Bania Aggarwal children have specifically high incidence of this disease. The reasons are not far to seek. For generation, Aggarwal banias have been a strictly vegetarian community. So are the social customs of the Hindus in South and to some extent in Bengal also. Most of these children come from rather affluent business families and their diets as per their standards and way of thinking were rather rich and good. But sadly diet lacked nutrition and was almost devoid of first class proteins. Sweets and rich fatty food was the staple diet of these families.

In other words proteins both qualitatively and quantitatively are essential for the proper upkeep of the liver. It has been well suggested that deficient diets such as are eaten by people in underdeveloped and Third World countries may have an indirect effect on the liver and not only produce certain changes in the liver in itself but also make it more prone to injuries by other noxius agents such as toxins, parasites and viruses. It is a very vicious circle. Once liver has been severely damaged, nutritional disturbances also occur because of defective intake of food as a result of loss of appetite, impaired digestion and lack of absorption of nutrients.

If proteins are good and essential for the liver then carbohydrates are equally essential for maintaining proper health of the liver. Liver plays an important role in glucose metabolism which is converted into glycogen and stored there. Until and unless adequate glycogen stores are available in the liver, it shall not be able to release more glucose into the blood from its glycogen stores. The liver utilises proteins for the process of formation of glucose to keep up its stores of glycogen whenever they became reduced by prolonged fasting or lack of carbohydrates in adequate amount. So, if instead of proper amounts of carbohydrate, excess of proteins are taken, they are going to be wasted from both viewpoints — body's need and for economic reasons. At the same time an unbalanced proportion of proteins and carbohydrates is not desirable. In other words, excess intake of proteins should not be taken on the false notion that they are good for the liver and at the same time ignoring the role of carbohydrates. Energy derived in this way from proteins is less efficiently used than that derived directly from the carbohydrates sources.

One cannot be more emphatic than to say that for maintaining the proper health of liver, expensive proteins in diet are not desirable since they are going to put strain on one's economic resources. Fats in adequate quantities coupled with vitamins and minerals should also be comprising important constituents of food.

Diet for the normal protection and maintenance of liver should be:

1. Nutritious and well-balanced, containing sufficient quantities of carbohydrates and proteins. Proteins in the diet should come both from animal and vegetable sources. In other words a balanced protein diet should be recommended. It may contain roughly combinations of bread, rice, cheese, meat, fish, curds, cereals and milk.

2. Fresh fruits like grapes, oranges, mosambi, papaya, mangoes, water melons, lichies, etc. are good source of natural sugars and are good for liver.
3. Rich spicy foods and excessive fats in the diets should be avoided. Pastries, cakes, sweets and chocolates, should be taken only in small quantities, and especially in growing children, adequate protein content of diet must be ensured.
4. Nutritional care of the patients with liver disease requires special attention and extra nutrition has to be supplemented to tide over the crisis. In a case of acute liver disease from any cause a good nourishing diet with high carbohydrate content has to be given and as soon as the person is recovering, in the convalescent stage adequate proteins have to be added.

In sum total, diet plays an important role in the causation of certain diseases of the liver and it assumes still greater significance when the liver is damaged and has to be sustained as well as protected.

ALCOHOL AND LIVER 3

Liver is one organ which bears the major brunt of alcohol abuse. The association of alcohol and major liver ailments is well known and there has been enough evidence to show that there is an inalienable link between the two. Fortunes of nations and its people have, to a large extent, been influenced by the degree of alcohol consumption of its people.

Alcohol has always been used as a form of social drink in the West and one which soothes the troubled mind, raising the spirits and giving energy. Alcoholic drinks are consumed against the false notion that they rejuvenate and bring strength to the individual. Such ideas were expressed succinctly by a writer of thirteenth century who wrote, "If alcoholic beverages sloweth age, it strengtheneth youth, it helpeth digestion; it abandoneth melancholia, it relisheth the heart, it lighteneth the mind, it quickeneth the spirits, it keepeth and preserveth the head from whirling, the eyes from dazzling, the tongue from lisping, the mouth from snaffling, the teeth from chattering and the throat from rattling: it keepeth the stomach from wambling, the heart from swelling, the hands from shivering, the sinews from shrinking, the veins from crumbling. It pries the bones from aching and the marrow from soaking". Fed on such thoughts, no wonder alcohol consumption has been on increase. Liquor is consumed in some societies at social get-together and festivities and is part of social milieu.

When one talks of effects of alcohol on liver one must differentiate between an occasional social drinker and a chronic regular drinker. An alcoholic individual has been described as one whose drinking causes him obvious difficulty physically, socially or in his marriage or occupation and who drinks more to overcome this difficulty. Such people become excessive drinkers, since their dependence upon alcohol has attained such a degree that it results in noticeable mental disturbance or in an interference with their bodily and mental health.

A certain group of people are more susceptible to consume more alcohol. Where alcoholic drinks are cheap it is the lower social class who are falling easy prey to it because of its easy availability. In our country because of cost, the weaker sections of society resort to consuming illicit and poor quality of beverages with the result that they are exposing themselves to more risks and health hazards. At one end of scale are poorer sections of society who are consuming inferior quality of alcohol coupled with poor intake of nutritious food because of economic factors while at the other end are the elite class, including business executives, busy professionals etc., who just do not know how to get away from the party circle. Some of them are addicted because of their social commitments while others are taking it to drown their loneliness. Alcohol consumption once started as a social obligation may subsequently become an addiction. Though occasional drink may not produce any bodily harm, yet often the question arises as to what quantity of alcohol is sufficient to produce liver injury and for how long.

The basic principle is that at least 24 hours must elapse before the next alcoholic bout to minimize the extent of liver injury. The steady imbiber of spirits is at much more risk than the 'spree' drinker though the total intake of alcohol may not be less in any of the two people. This is because the person .who takes his drinks intermittently gives his liver rest and a chance to repair itself but this is not so in a regular who is exposing his liver daily to some level of injury. There are no safe limits to which alcohol may be consumed. A rough estimate puts 60g of spirit in men and a mere 20g in women to be safe levels. There is no doubt that alcohol even consumed in small quantities but regularly over long periods is going to produce liver damage. It has been calculated that about 190g of alcohol consumed daily for 10 years can result in the production of alcoholic cirrhosis. But there are no hard and fast rules. If large quantities of alcohol are consumed daily without much interval in between, only short time shall be required to produce the damage.

Basically heavy drinker has been classified as one whose daily consumption of pure alcohol exceeds 0.1 litre. Such people are definitely going to show the ill effects of alcohol and that too at an early stage.

Liver disease is a major chronic illness among at least 4-5 million American citizens suffering from alcoholism. There is enough evidence to show that in two-thirds of alcoholics who drink enough wine, beer or whisky to interfere with food intake, social and work responsibility their liver suffers and not less than 10 to 30% of these people develop cirrhosis of liver. Alcoholic cirrhosis is the fourth commonest cause of death in United States. Similar figures indicating liver damage due to alcohol are also available from the other western countries.

Whenever and wherever the consumption of alcohol has been excessive in a community or a country there has been steep rise in the incidence of liver injury due to alcohol leading to cirrhosis. The reverse side of the picture is also true. During war time when wine was rationed in France there was substantial reduction in mortality from alcoholic liver disease but it rose dramatically in the period immediately following war and so did the amount of alcohol consumption. There is enough evidence from morbidity and mortality studies to show the physical health hazards produced by heavy alcohol consumption. Alcoholic cirrhosis is one of the major causes of death in middle aged persons in many countries of the world.

Regular and continued consumption of alcohol either as wine or spirits leads to liver damage. Even a single large dose of alcohol given to healthy volunteers can produce significant liver injury. Alcohol given in fairly large doses (200g) daily for 18 days to healthy human volunteers showed fatty changes in the liver and change in the ultra-structures of liver cells.

What happens when alcohol is taken? Alcohol is absorbed into the blood stream without a thing called digestion. It enters partly from the stomach and a large portion from the intestines. Absorption of alcohol, to a large extent, is controlled by the fact whether it is taken on an empty stomach or mixed with carbonated drinks as both these situations shall hasten its absorption and quick effects. Whatever be the effects on the nervous system and other systems of the body, it is the liver which bears a major thrust of its ill effects. Since 90 to 95% of it is being oxidized in the liver.

Many lay people consider alcohol as a nutrient little realising that though it produces energy yet it has little in common with other energy rich compounds like carbohydrates and fats which can be effectively utilized and stored in the body. While alcohol is basically foreign to the body, it cannot be stored effectively and to a large extent is to be disposed of by the body by the process of oxidization in which liver plays the major role.

Liver is involved in the process of converting glucose into glycogen and vice versa. If an individual drinks and does not eat properly, there may be no dietary carbohydrates and thus the body fails in its mechanism of maintaining glycogen stores. This interferes with the normal process of maintaining blood glucose levels and very low blood sugar levels have been produced due to the disturbance of liver metabolism by alcohol and even death may result. In an alcoholic even the drugs taken for any purpose shall not act adequately as their metabolism in the liver shall be interfered with.

Alcohol cannot be stored, since it is wholly being metabolized. A healthy individual cannot use more than 160-180 g of alcohol per day.

It is said that alcoholics run on spirits, since one gram of alcohol shall give rise to seven calories but these are only empty calories. They really provide no nutrition. It is a very false notion amongst people that alcohol provides them the real kick and that is why they go on talking it ad lib. The duration and amount of alcohol consumed shall, to a large extent, determine the development of liver damage. The damage being produced in the liver is as a result of oxidation products of alcohol which accumulate in the liver and produce toxic injury.

A number of factors may be operative in the production of liver injury. Before one remarks on the sequence of events that take place in a person who is taking alcohol, one should differentiate between the occasional drinker and heavy drinker. In the first category is a person who takes a peg or two and follows it up with good nutrient food, the chances of his or her developing permanent liver damage are low, since liver cells shall be able to withstand the injury and regenerate themselves. But the ill effects start in those who are consuming large amount of alcohol everyday for a number of years. It is here that the nutrition of the liver cells suffers and irreparable damage may be done.

In the early stages, the liver is enlarged because of fatty change, since every liver cell is laden with fat. This is the earliest stage and is called the fatty liver. It is as a result of enhanced synthesis and reduced oxidation of fatty acids derived from dietary fat. Luckily this condition of liver is reversible if the patient stops drinking and takes a well-balanced nutritious food. Liver is enlarged but smooth to feel. The person complains of indigestion, dyspepsia, belching and loss of appetite. If the person abstains completely from alcohol at this stage, it generally takes about 4 to 12 weeks for the liver to come back to its normal size and the first evidence of normalcy may be improvement in appetite.

But if the drinking is not stopped despite the early warnings the patient gradually passes on to the stage of inflammation of liver (Hepatitis). The liver cells show degenerative changes in their cell structure and there is abnormal functional impairment. Alcoholic hepatitis is a serious ailment and may prove fatal. It is a true inflammatory response in the liver which occurs in 10 to 20 per cent of alcoholics especially when there is an abrupt increase in their consumption of alcohol. Patient may suffer nausea, vomiting, weakness, weight loss, abdominal pain, fever, diarrhoea and jaundice, etc. The patient looks ill with a characteristic earthen colored face and pronounced fever. When liver enlarges suddenly, it causes severe pain though it is soft and rounded. Some patients may bleed from the stomach as a result of gastritis or because of extensive liver damage.

At this stage liver function tests may not reveal the true serious nature of the underlying disease. There are raised levels of enzymes with fall in albumin and rise in gamma globulin levels. Liver biopsy shall show liver cells which are completely replaced by fat and there are areas of necrosis and inflammatory cells.

Alcoholic hepatitis is a serious complication and death may occur in great majority of people at this stage. Main differentiation of this stage is from viral hepatitis which sometimes may be difficult to differentiate except that the history of chronic alcohol intake shall point towards the probable impression of alcoholic liver disease.

Those who survive from alcoholic hepatitis, at least half of them ultimately pass on to cirrhosis which is the last stage of alcoholic injury to the liver and resembles other types of end stage liver injury.

But it looks very ambiguous to say that every alcoholic does not develop cirrhosis. Samuel Johnson said "One may drink wine and be nothing the worse for it; in another wine may have effects so inflammatory as to injure him both in body and mind". It only means that not everyone who drinks excessively develops liver damage, since a number of chronic alcoholics have been found to have normal livers. Only one in twelve persons who are chronic heavy drinkers, develops cirrhosis. This paradox has been explained on the basis that liver injury in alcoholics is genetically determined.

There is no doubt that cirrhosis and alcohol are closely associated. Development of cirrhosis in alcoholics may be due to an inborn defect in liver metabolism and is specific for that person. A number of factors ranging from formation of fibrous and collagen tissue, immunological hyperactivity, hypermetabolic state and nutrition have been incriminated in the production of alcoholic cirrhosis.

Cirrhosis is a slow and stealthy killer which may take years to show itself but when it does, the damage has already been done and probably it is point of no return.

Nutrition vis-à-vis alcohol and cirrhosis has a very important role to play. Chronic alcoholics are usually suffering from malnutrition. Reasons are obvious, since some of them do not take adequate amount of nutrition as their appetites are poor and they are also left with little money to buy the high protein nutritious diet. Whatsoever little they are left with is being spent on alcohol.

Excessive alcohol intake affects normal diet patterns so that nutrition of the liver cells suffers. Alcoholics suffer from lowered absorption of vitamin B complex especially vitamin B_1 and B_6 as compared to healthy non-alcoholic subjects. This is as a result of inability to absorb these specific vitamins from food. Similarly low levels of zinc and magnesium have been associated with alcohol consumption. Thus one finds an all-round interference with the absorption of nutrients.

There are studies which show that alcohol and not an inadequate diet is the cause of cirrhosis. This calls into question the value of trying to prevent cirrhosis in alcoholics merely by giving them good diets. Though alcoholism contributes in a great measure to cirrhosis, yet it is not clear as to how much of the disease per se is due to alcohol and how much due to an inadequate diet.

More than twenty years ago Dr. Lieber and his colleagues from New York had found that fatty liver, the most benign state of cirrhosis could be produced in volunteers given alcohol with adequate dietary intake. Question remained whether alcoholic hepatitis and cirrhosis could also be directly linked to alcohol ingestion rather than to deficient diets.

This problem could not be studied in volunteers in view of the severity of the damage involved. And animals were not willing to consume enough alcohol to produce damage when the alcohol was given as part of the drinking water. This problem was solved by incorporating alcohol in totally liquid diets.

Specifically they gave 15 baboons totally liquid diets that contained adequate nutrients and 50 per cent of the animals caloric needs in alcohol. The baboons remained on this diet for an average of 15 months. During this time they developed the sequential stages of liver damage seen in human alcoholics. All developed fatty liver, five progressed to hepatitis and five progressed still further to cirrhosis. These findings have major implications and that is that we cannot prevent cirrhosis in the alcoholics merely by controlling the diet.

A person taking alcohol must understand that he cannot go on taking alcohol under the false sense of security that if he takes good protein diet along with alcohol, his liver shall not suffer any ill effects. On the other hand, if an alcoholic stops taking alcohol, his liver shall not show any improvement if his diet is not nutritious and well-balanced, since the integrity of liver cells depends to a large extent on the high level of proteins and nutrients in the diet.

Another interesting study where the alcohol intake and dietary habits of 304 alcoholic, hospitalized patients was studied appears to be quite revealing. There were 195 patients with liver cirrhosis, 40 in early stages of cirrhosis and 69 patients without cirrhosis. Dietary intakes were assessed for a period of at least 2 years before the presenting illness and alcohol contributed 50 to 58 per cent of total calories during this time. Two-thirds of the patients drank excessively for more than 20 years. The diets of both cirrhotic and non-cirrhotic patients were poor when judged by traditional standards. There was all-round deficiency in the quality of diet. However, non-cirrhotic had somewhat higher protein and caloric intakes from food than did the cirrhotic, suggesting that poor nutrition did play a role along with the direct toxic effects of alcohol in the development of severe liver disease.

A number of factors play their part. It is not only inadequate and poor quality of diet but also lack of appetite as well as non-absorption of nutrients from the gastrointestinal tract. The role of deficient and poor diets cannot be minimized, since most of the alcoholics have had poor intake of nutritious food. It is also well accepted that dietary deficiencies adversely affect the survival of an alcoholic.

Once cirrhosis has developed, it is an irreversible stage to some extent. The liver from its enlarged state starts shrinking. The liver is divided into small regular uniformly distributed lobules by fibrous septa until it assumes a nodular appearance. The fat content of liver decreases and the liver has now shrunk to such level that the cause of cirrhosis cannot be detected. In later years a macronodular cirrhosis develops after the patient becomes an abstainer and active regeneration of the liver becomes possible.

But every alcoholic developing cirrhosis of liver need not necessarily pass through the stage of fatty liver and hepatitis. When there is fully developed cirrhosis there is fluid in the abdomen (ascites), enlarged parotid glands, atrophy of testes and prominence of breasts (Gynaecomastia) in men. Person gets wasted but has a protruding abdomen and swollen legs with a tendency to bleed. Muscle mass gets less. There is loss of memory, insomnia, irritability, hallucinations and tremors as the disease progresses. Some of the cirrhotics bleed from the rupture of dilated blood vessels in the food pipe (oesophageal varices) and this is a serious emergency which may prove life-threatening. Once a full picture of cirrhosis develops the life span may not be more than 3-4 years. Most of the cirrhotics die either of intercurrent infections, bleeds or liver failure.

Question arises as to how to assess liver involvement in alcoholics. It may be a very silent process which damages the liver relentlessly. Naturally a number of factors have to be gone into to look at the extent of liver damage in an alcoholic with a long history of abuse.

There is often history of loss of appetite, weight loss in early stages. Some people may come complaining of pain in the upper abdomen on right side. Liver function tests may not be deranged in early stages. A number of enzymes are estimated (AST, ALT) which are raised, indicating liver injury. Serum glutamate dehydrogenase is a reliable indicator of liver cell necrosis in alcoholics and so is alkaline phosphatase which is markedly raised in alcoholic hepatitis. But surprisingly, very sensitive biochemical tests may fail to reveal liver damage due to alcohol and for this the doctors have to resort to a simple procedure like liver biopsy. It is important, since it shall confirm the presence or absence of liver damage and as to the stage of liver injury. Interestingly at a certain stage of liver injury in the alcoholic, the whole process can be reversed especially if the person can overcome his addiction and is taken off it, coupled with the use of a good nourishing diet.

It is very important that ill effects of alcohol on liver are recognised early. Most of the times the alcoholic complains of loss of appetite, nausea coming in the early hours of the morning, right upper abdominal pain and dyspepsia. Some people are brought because of social problems. A few complain of tremors, depression and remorsefulness.

Liver in such cases is enlarged and painful. There may be other signs of liver failure. Biochemical tests like raised enzyme levels when present are helpful in making an impression of liver injury but when normal even then do not rule out liver injury. Alcoholic hepatitis is a more serious condition, and is often brought on particularly after a heavy bout of drinking, vomiting, diarrhoea or acute infection. There is fever, yellowness of eyes (jaundice) and behaviour disturbances. Person may be vomiting repeatedly. Signs of liver damage and nutritional deficiency are present.

Cirrhosis tends to improve slowly. When portal hypertension has already developed, alcohol abstinence cannot now reverse the process, because the damage has already been done and there is hardly any benefit which the patient can drive by the wheel turning back. Alcoholic hepatitis takes quite a long time to recover and may persist for number of years, the patient sitting on the edge of a volcano waiting to erupt if exposure to alcohol abuse is continued and then we have at our hands a cirrhotic rather than a hepatitis with poor prognosis.

The most important issue is how to prevent injury to liver from alcohol. As said earlier, there can be nothing better than avoidance of alcoholic drinks. But in this present age of high-living people are exposed to a certain milieu and society where alcoholic drinks and spirits form a very essential part of daily living, the best advice is to be moderate with your drinks. Take drinks where alcoholic content is low. Do not take more than one to two pegs at a time and to minimize liver injury take alcohol infrequently and not at regular intervals. This gives time for the liver to regenerate and recover.

Anybody who takes alcoholic drinks must supplement his diet with adequate amounts of high class proteins, and supplementary vitamins of B complex group. Though the role of diet in the prevention of liver injury in alcoholics is disputed, yet one cannot deny the fact that diet has an inalienable role to play.

This advice is for those who take an occasional drink and where there is no evidence of any untoward liver damage.

For those with evidence of liver injury, they must abstain from alcohol forever and the care of the person instituted under a properly qualified physician.

A process of detoxification should be instituted once the patient is taken off alcohol. To start with, intravenous infusions of glucose and vitamins are given, followed by fruit juices and high calorie foods. Appetite of such patients is generally poor but gradually returns as the liver injury regresses.

The person has to be taken away from the previous environment and social milieu. Some of the alcoholics are untrustworthy and may make very wild promises to look after their family, job and social obligations. These promises should not be taken on their face value and even a psychiatric help or that of Alcoholic's Anonymous may be needed.

The alcoholic has to be treated with adequate bed rest, nutritious diet supplemented with vitamins, etc. For complications like liver failure, psychiatric disturbances the best judge is the treating physician.

Lastly, it must be impressed on the alcoholic that if he wants to improve the quality of life, he must abstain from alcohol for all times to come. Abstentin must be complete and total, since if the liver is subjected to repeated injuries the process of regeneration will subsequently fail. Similarly an alcoholic liver is more sensitive and may not react to some drugs in the same way as a normal healthy liver shall, so one must take precautions in the use of certain drugs like sedatives, analgesics (paracetamol), etc.

In the end, one must emphasize that alcohol does damage the liver and is going to produce certain level of injury which at a certain stage may not be reversible and the consequences of it may be disastrous for the alcoholic.

Alcohol Abuse: Some Facts

1. Alcohol abuse may occur in families due to a genetic predisposition so those with a strong family history of alcoholism must avoid it lest they become chronic alcoholics.
2. Women do not tolerate alcohol as well as those of men since they lack an enzyme which breaks it. Result, women get intoxicated earlier than men.
3. One alcoholic drink is equivalent to one ounce of hard liquor, six ounces of wine and 12 ounces of beer.
4. Absorption of alcohol from the stomach is delayed by food especially fatty foods. Alcohol taken with carbonated drinks is absorbed more rapidly as compared to water which makes its absorption slower.
5. An average liver oxidises alcohol at the rate of one-third or one-half ounce per hour, which means if three large pegs of whisky are taken it shall take at least three hours before it is completely removed from the blood stream.
6. More than two drinks per day put load on the liver. If a person takes alcohol faster than the rate at which body can dispose it, the harmful effects accumulate over a period of time.
7. Prolonged drinking adversely affects all systems of the body. Liver bears the major brunt. Fatty liver is the first stage of damage characterized by loss of appetite, morning nausea and vague pain in liver area.

   This is followed by a more serious form of liver damage—Alcoholic Hepatitis. It develops in people who have been consuming alcohol heavily for more than two years. Here there is not only loss of appetite, fever but also jaundice. Last and final stage of liver damage is alcoholic cirrhosis where there is swelling of abdomen, feet and marked weakness.

8. Besides liver damage in men who drink heavily, there are chances of developing cancer of the mouth, food pipe, stomach and rectum.
9. There is no safe limit of drinking. People who drink occasionally have less chance of liver injury, since they give their liver time to repair. It is the regular imbiber of alcohol who is at maximum risk.

YELLOW PERIL

4

Of all the liver problems jaundice is one with which every lay person is familiar and the very appearance of it creates a sense of apprehension about its ill effects. No wonder in the lay language it is called 'Yellow Peril'. The words 'Icterus' and 'Jaundice' are interchangeable, the former deriving from Neo-Latin taken from Greek and the latter from the French word 'Jaunde'. They both mean 'Yellow' and refer to the characteristic coloring of the body especially of the skin, white of the eye and mucous surfaces. There is peculiar yellowish or greenish staining of the body and the person gives an earthen yellow appearance. A person gets jaundiced when there is excess of bile pigment (bilirubin) in the blood.

Whenever a person gets jaundiced the first thoughts which come to mind are that of hepatitis, little realising that there can be innumerable diseases responsible for it. Jaundice is often the first and sometimes the only indication of the liver disease. But it is a mere symptom and may occur in most diseases of the liver.

Very often the presence of jaundice may not be observed for a number of days either because of seeing it in poor light or the symptoms are so mild that the person just ignores them. Quite commonly a family member or friend observes it or the sufferer may start feeling out of sorts or observe that his urine has got rather high dark colour.

Jaundice can occur in numerous ways. Normally bilirubin is being metabolised, synthesized and excreted in a way that its levels remain within normal limits. It is its abnormal levels leading to accumulation, which gives rise to jaundice. Let us have a look at the various ways in which jaundice can be seen.

(a) Excessive bilirubin is produced in the body when red cells are being destroyed at an abnormally rapid rate and the resulting bile pigment is more than what a normal liver can handle. This is called haemolytic type of jaundice. Common examples of this are congenital haemolytic jaundice, sickle cell anaemia, Rh incompatibility, incompatible blood transfusion and excessive haemolysis resulting due to severe infections (malaria, viral) drugs, poisons and severe burns.

(b) Hepatocellular jaundice where the bilirubin production is normal but the capacity of the liver to utilise it (conjugation and excretion) is itself hampered due to liver cell dysfunction which may be due to infection, inflammation or any disease which involves the liver itself. This is the type of jaundice seen in infective hepatitis, yellow fever, severe bacterial infections, cirrhosis and diseases directly affecting the liver.

(c) Obstructive jaundice: In this, though there is no liver cell dysfunction and the amount of bilirubin produced is normal, yet there exists an obstruction to the normal passage of it in reaching the intestines with the result that bilirubin regurgitates into the blood stream and its levels rise. Obstructive jaundice may be due either to intrahepatic obstruction or outside the liver in the biliary passages. Examples of former are congenital defects, cholangitis (infections, drugs) and the latter due to stones, tumours or strictures.

These are some of the common causes of jaundice, but then again jaundice per se is not a disease but symptomatic of an underlying disorder and this is the primary disease which has to be looked into.

The degree of jaundice shall not determine the complaints the patient has. In cases of jaundice due to hepatocellular dysfunction it is the symptoms of hepatic disease which shall predominate while in obstructive jaundice the picture is more of pain due to stones. Apart from yellow staining of the skin, jaundice may cause no symptoms. A patient with deep jaundice due to cancer of the pancreas (sweet bread) may be rather in well state as compared to a patient of hepatocellular jaundice where degree of jaundice is less but the patient is more ill. In other words, jaundice itself does not produce any major impairment of health.

Let us take into consideration some of the causes operative in a case of jaundice which can very often be assessed by the sufferer himself. The familial occurrence of jaundice should suggest the possibility of it being congenital hyperbilirubinemia, hepatitis and gall stones.

Occupation of the patient is important particularly with special reference to exposure to hepatotoxic agents. If a person is working in brewery, hotel or bar where wine/alcoholic drinks are easily available it shall point to the alcohol as an aetiological factor. Similarly paramedical staff (nurses and technicians) who work in hospitals, blood banks where they are working in the process of drawing or administering blood or administering injections etc., the danger of puncturing their fingers and contracting hepatitis are very much there.

Contact of the person with jaundiced patients is also of importance especially in nurseries, hostels, camps, schools and hospitals where hepatitis is common. Similarly during an epidemic of jaundice the diagnosis is not difficult.

If the patient has had any injection or blood transfusion in the preceding six months, the diagnosis of hepatitis (serum/ hepatitis B) is very probable. This can also occur if the patient has had blood drawn out for any blood tests or had himself vaccinated or tattooed or was subjected to dental treatment.

Some drugs are also known to produce jaundice. So this should always be kept in mind. Of the commonly used drugs, one may mention here isoniazid (anti-tubercular drug) male sex hormones and oral contraceptives.

Age of the person suffering from jaundice is important in reaching at the aetiological factor. If jaundice appears during the first week of life in a new born child, it may be due to normal physiology and is called physiological jaundice which is usually mild, attains maximum levels by the second or third day and fades away by the end of first week.

If the jaundice in the infant gets prolonged then the factor of pre-maturity, Rh-incompatibility and sepsis with infection from umbilicus should be considered. Any infant who develops deep jaundice within the first twenty-four hours Rh incompatibility should be looked into and the parents investigated.

In an infant developing jaundice later on congenital obliteration of the bile ducts, sickle cell anaemia, hereditary spherocytosis and even neonatal hepatitis are some of the factors.

A fat, middle aged female is more likely to suffer from gall stones. Similarly cancer of liver and gall bladder incidence increases as the age advances. Drug-induced jaundice shall be uncommon in infants and young children.

If a patient has been complaining of dyspepsia and intolerance to fatty foods again the pointer is towards gall stones. Similarly if jaundice has appeared after surgery, trauma of the biliary tract or stricture should be the likely cause. If a person has been having progressive failure of health, weight loss, abdominal discomfort and loss of appetite during the preceding few months carcinoma of the biliary tract, pancreas of liver be considered.

If one really analyses the complaints and symptoms of the patient rather diligently, lot of information can be gained. The way the person started with his illness is equally important. If the patient experienced nausea, loss of appetite, aversion to smoking, ill health during the preceding week or so before jaundice came, it is more suggestive of viral hepatitis. The presence of symptoms of abdominal disorder for several months accompanied by weight loss will be a pointer towards malignancy. Skin of a jaundiced patient may show bleeding spots which shall be in favour of hepatocellular damage. In obstructive jaundice, there may be scratch marks indicative of pruritis. This is also seen in cholestatic form of infective hepatitis.

Colour of jaundice is equally important in making an impression about the type of jaundice. It is of mild yellow colour in haemolytic jaundice, orange coloured in hepatocellular variety and deep greenish in obstructive variety. Presence of fluid in abdomen and loss of secondary sexual characters shall favour cirrhosis.

It is interesting to note that very simple common day observations shall help in differentiating about the probable cause of jaundice. Urine shall become dark coloured (some call it looking like tea or coca cola) for several days preceding the appearance of jaundice in hepatitis and as the disease process improves, the colour shall revert towards normal. Stools shall be clay coloured indicative of biliary obstruction. A person having brown stools with deep jaundice means having hepatocellular jaundice. A sensible advice to the patient is to look at his urine and stools daily and record their colour. Fluctuations in colour of these products shall be a good guide to the improvement or otherwise of the person.

In any patient of jaundice, since the aetiological factors are multiple, a number of investigations are required to make the correct diagnosis. These are in addition to a carefully taken history and physical examination done by physician with a view to assess the presence of liver enlargement, fluid in the abdomen, evidence of scratch marks on the skin, colour of the type of jaundice, any glands either in the body or abdomen as well as presence of gall bladder mass or lump. Assessment of mental functions like intellectual deterioration, disturbances of sleep rhythm is equally important in a case of jaundice since any deviation from the normal personality traits in such people shall favour the development of hepatic failures.

Early recognition of hepatic failure is important, since late diagnosis means poor prognosis. In addition to history and examination, number of tests are done to confirm the diagnosis of the underlying condition. The wide range of tests include urine examination (for the presence or absence of bile salts, pigments and urobilinogen), white cell count (raised count excludes viral hepatitis but favours toxic hepatitis, alcoholic hepatitis, cholangitis, neoplasm, etc.), Comob's test, blood fragility (to diagnose haemolysis), serum bilirubin (to assess the degree of jaundice), enzymes like SGOT, SGPT (rise in liver dysfunction and hepatitis). Alkaline phosphatase (double the normal levels favour neoplasm) and other tests of liver function.

But the liver tests are of limited value and have to be looked in the light of full clinical profile. Ultrasound and X-ray of the abdomen may show gall stones. Barium study shall be helpful in cancer pancreas. Other specialised tests include needle biopsy of liver, ERCP (endoscopic retrograde cholangiogiopancreatography) percutaneous transhepatic cholangiography and peritonoscopy. All the tests and investigative procedures have to be carried by the physician in charge, depending on as to how the patient is to be managed.

Depending on the diagnosis of the basic disease, the treatment shall be instituted which may be medical or even surgical. But all shall depend on the correct diagnosis. To quote Nellis B. Foster, 'For the most brilliant discoveries in therapeutics or the most skilled surgery avail nothing if the patients' disease is not correctly diagnosed.'

Now let us look at a very common condition which goes almost synonymous with jaundice according to lay terminology and this is viral hepatitis, variously termed infective or infection hepatitis, epidemic hepatitis, serum hepatitis, post transfusion hepatitis, etc.

Viral hepatitis may be defined as a form of systemic viral infection accompanied by hepatic cell inflammation and necrosis with a characteristic clinical picture. It is of worldwide distribution. In majority of the people, the disease runs a mild course. Distinct three viral agents are known to produce the acute inflammation of liver. Though these viruses (hepatitis A, hepatitis B and non-A, non-B hepatitis) are distinct in their characteristics, yet the basic pathology of liver in all these is the same. The recorded history of viral hepatitis finds its origins in accounts which date way back to ancient times. First mention of this scourage was in Talmud: Armies lost battles because of this disease and often it was labelled as camp jaundice. Wars have been the worst periods when the disease is at its peak. It shall not be difficult to understand this situation in view of the prevailing low standards of hygiene and inadequate water supply at the time of war. Important wars where hepatitis had its toll were during American Civil War, Napoleon's campaign in Egypt, British Army in Flanders in 1743 and subsequently in Germany between 1761-63. Over 70,000 cases of jaundice were reported among union army troops during the Civil War (1861-1865). Similarly epidemics of jaundice with high mortality occurred in the Franco-Prussian War of 1870, the Boer War in South Africa, the Russo-Japanese War of 1904-1906 and during both World-Wars I and II. Though in olden times the morbidity and mortality due to hepatitis was very high, almost foretelling the fortunes of nations yet even in present age, wars have been places of onslaught of hepatitis. A glaring example is Korean War and Vietnam War where once again epidemics of jaundice raged havoc.

Epidemics of hepatitis during peace time occur infrequently and that too in a small scale. Institutions like Camps, Jails, Hostels, Schools, Hospitals, etc. often fall prey to it, but then the morbidity is not very high. Probably the biggest epidemic in recorded history in civil population occurred in Delhi in the year 1955, when following floods and diversion of the river Yamuna, the water supply of Delhi was contaminated with sewerage. The result was an estimate of 35 to 40 thousand people who fell victim to it.

But then natural calamities like floods, disasters bring the epidemics, since there is little control over the sanitary measures in large scale collection of people in relief camps.

How the infection spreads: The spread of hepatitis (type A) is mainly through faeco oral route and a number of common sources of infection are identified: contaminated water supplies, infected food and its handlers, sewerage contaminated food and eating of raw unclean foods, including sea food.

Drinking water is frequently contaminated at the source like when people defile the water supply reservoirs with their ablutions, etc. Other way is when the drinking water gets contaminated with sewerage water due to faulty drainage. Direct contamination of food is a very important mode of infection. This usually happens when an infected person serves food or touches plates, glasses, etc. with unclean hands. In fact cooks and bearers in hotels, clubs and homes who have suffered from attack of hepatitis in the recent past should not be allowed either to cook the food or handle it.

It would be educative to recount some of the important case histories. In early 1968, in Michigan, sixty-one cases of hepatitis occurred in young persons in the age group of 10-19 years. Since the cases occurred in a community amongst youngsters, investigations were carried out to find common source of infection. Investigations revealed that in a local bakery, one of the employees directly involved in the baking of pastries had had an illness of hepatitis one month before the outbreak and since this man had handled these foods, the icing of the pastries acted as the vehicle of infection.

There are numerous instances where minor epidemics have been traced to cafeteria and eating shops. In Minneapolis, 107 cases of hepatitis. A were traced primarily to consumption of cold sandwiches served in a departmental store restaurant and prepared by a person who had suffered the disease.

In the West, where seafood is considered a delicacy—wherever clams grown in polluted water are consumed, hepatitis results. Ingestion of raw shell fish and steamed clams is an important factor. Unfortunately steaming does not kill the hepatitis virus in the gastrointestinal tract of the clam. This is one occasion where cook books of gourmets have erred. They advise ingestion soon after the shell opens when the internal temperature in the clam is not very high as the meat at this stage is soft and delicious. For the destruction of hepatitis virus the heat required is in such amount that it is likely to toughen the meat.

Estimates of the incidence of hepatitis following eating of raw shell fish and other sea food, though is not very high, yet it does require caution amongst communities where the incidence of hepatitis itself is not very high.

Similarly use of human sewage for soil fertilization can result in frozen fruit related epidemics. Though direct contact with infected persons and water supply are the main culprits in the spread of type-A hepatitis, the main mode of spread of serum hepatitis (hepatitis-B) is by parenteral route. This is the major mode of spread when infected serum contaminated syringes, needles or instruments are used for injection, inoculations and transfusions. Use of unsterile instruments for dental treatment, ear-piercing, manicure, acupuncture, tattooing and vaccination are significant modes of spreading the infection. Thus epidemics of hepatitis-B occurred after smallpox vaccination and similarly after yellow fever inoculations. Blood transfusions remain a very important source of transmission, especially if due attention is not paid to the proper screening of blood donors. Such episodes are very common when blood is used from commercial or paid donors. Interestingly type-B hepatitis spreads not only by the blood and its products but also through semen and saliva. Homosexuals are at risk of contracting hepatitis and particularly the number of their sexual contacts become an important means of spreading the infection. A mother who is carrier of hepatitis-B, transmits the infection to the child at the time of birth and during subsequent close contact. Inter-family spread may also occur and this may be by kissing, use of same utensils, tooth brushes and razors.

Very interesting observations were made in Scandinavian countries where hepatitis has been transmitted in Swedish track finders due to scratches sustained during the cross country races. The added factor of communal washing and close contact also played its part.

Drug addicts are very prone to suffer from it, since they use unsterile syringes and in vast majority the same syringe is being used by the other members of the commune without taking adequate precautions. Hospital staff (doctors, nurses and other paramedical staff) who are in close contact with such patients and their blood run greater risk of contracting hepatitis. It is equally so in dialysis units or open heart surgery units where repeated blood transfusions have to be given.

Attendants and hospital staff may contract the disease by coming in contact with the infected blood either through pricking or through abrasious or cuts in their skins. Similarly, Dental surgeons when operating on hepatitis-B carrier persons (HbsAg) are equally at risk either by holes in their gloves or cuts. In brief, parenteral route is the main mode of spread of type-B hepatitis.

Carrier rates as high as 20% of the virus have been reported from some parts of the world, though on average the carrier state is between 10-15%. Just like type-B hepatitis, non-A, non-B hepatitis spreads mainly through blood transfusions and accounts for the mode of spread in more than 75% of the people. Cases have also been reported where non-A, non-B hepatitis was transmitted with drug abuse, and in renal transplant recipients. The mode of spread is as in hepatitis-B. Oral infectivity and faecal spread of this virus is not anticipated.

Summing up, percutaneous transmission of hepatitis-B and non-A, non-B viral hepatitis is characteristic of these two forms of hepatitis, though it is not observed in type-A hepatitis.

What is the organism?

Hepatitis is caused by a small virus which is extremely small and can evade the smallest of filters, since it is only 25 to 28th millionth of a millimeter. The virus of hepatitis-A is smaller than that of hepatitis-B (42 millionth of a millimeter) and the virus of non-A, non-B hepatitis is in size intermediate between the two. Hepatitis virus is RNA virus whereas hepatitis-B virus is a DNA virus.

The virus of hepatitis-A can be identified in the stools of patient's from about two weeks till one week after the appearance of jaundice. A serum antibody (anti-HAV) appears as the patient's stools become negative for virus and is detected in faeces of the person for a number of years. Non-human primates like chimpanzees and marmosets (small South African monkeys) are susceptible to hepatitis-A virus.

The virus is heat resistant but heavy chlorination and boiling for 15minutes can deactivate the virus. Interestingly carrier state which means chronic infection and an epidemiological source of infection has not been documented in hepatitis-A infection.

Hepatitis-B virus is a tiny 42 mm size spherical DNA virus. Three types of particles have been seen under the electron microscope. The complex Dane particle is the complete hepatitis-B virus (HBV). An antigen first detected in an Australian aborigin and present on the surface of hepatitis-B virus, is termed hepatitis-B surface antigen (HbSAg). It appears in the blood about six weeks after infection and disappears by three months. If it persists for more than six months it means that the patient is now going to be in a chronic carrier state. Chimpanzees have been infected with this virus but no other non-human primate including monkeys or marmosets can be infected. Carrier state which results in more than 10% of sufferers from this disease portends bad for sufferers from it. Interestingly men are six times more likely to become carriers as compared to women. Why this sex differentiation is not explainable. A virus distinct from hepatitis-A and hepatitis-B was identified as being responsible for causing hepatitis. The earliest evidence suggesting the agent was the observation of episodes of viral hepatitis that could not be attributed either to HAV/HBV or to other recognised agents. This agent has been transmitted to Chimpanzees who show a mild antibody response. It is said that the picture of a case of non-A, non-B hepatitis shall closely resemble that of type-B though in a modified form.

How do sufferers of hepatitis present?

The commonest mode of infection in viral hepatitis is oral faecal spread. Blood or stools may contain the virus in high concentration even when the person is not having any symptoms and signs. The presence of virus means setting stage for the spread of the disease and the virus gains entry into the body through contaminated food or water. Once inside the body it incubates for 3 days to 3 weeks during which it multiplies in the intestinal lining and then invades the liver through the blood stream.

The commonest age group most susceptible to suffer is children and young adults. The disease has a milder course in younger age group and the incidences decrease with advancing age. It only mcans that with advancing age, body acquires immunity. The severity of the infection is related both to the virulence of the organism and the population at risk. Thus under-nutrition, alcoholism and pre-existing liver damage shall make the person suffer from a more serious profile.

Serum hepatitis, on the other hand, mainly spread by parenteral inoculation and the faeces of sufferers are not inflective.

The incubation period of the virus in the body ranges from 6 weeks to 6 months. It has a more insidious course as compared to the type-A hepatitis which is more acute and severe. Hepatitis-B occurs at all ages and there is no decrease in susceptibility with advancing years. The clinical presentation and pathology in hepatitis-A, B and non-A, non-B hepatitis is basically the same except for the severity, route of infection and subsequent course of events.

The basic lesion is acute inflammation of the liver. The liver cells show necrosis along with presence of inflammatory cells. The centres of the liver lobules show maximum involvement but the reticule in framework is usually well preserved. This acts as a form of basic structure where liver cells regenerate from outwards and complete the full cycle of repair.

As the acute inflammation subsides, the liver starts recovering towards it path of normalcy. The inflammatory cells now disappear and the process of cleaning up starts.

Rarely the inflammation may be so massive that the whole lobule of liver may be involved. Liver gets shrunken, is flaccid and a lobe may show severe degree of atrophy. Those who survive, nodules may form. The cut surface may show a nutmeg appearance with collapse of reticulin network. More often it is followed by scar formation. Further continuation of this process gives rise to chronic persistent hepatitis. A further stage of this process where necrosis in portal zones enlarges and they become irregular with extension of septa into the lobules is called Chronic Active Hepatitis. Classically a case of hepatitis has got three phases:

1. Pre-icteric (pre-jaundice)
2. Jaundice (icteric stage)
3. Convalescent or recovery stage.

Pre-icteric or pre-jaundice stage: This is the stage when the virus can be detected in the faeces and blood before the tell-tale yellow appears in the patient's eyes and skin. It is also the period when the person is in the maximum infective stage shedding infection constantly. It lasts from three to nine days, and now viraemia is maximal. The earliest and most constant symptom is loss of appetite. The very thought of food may be unwelcome. Patient can take his breakfast with quite relish and as the day passes the appetite decreases and by night he develops almost total aversion to food. There is total loss of desire to smoke and a smoker notices it quite to his chagrin. Nausea, vomiting, slight to moderate fever, general malaise in the form of aches and pains, abdominal discomfort and constipation are present. Person may complain of a dull ache sometimes leading to severe pain in the upper part of abdomen on right side. This is indicative of liver enlargement and this pain in liver is further increased either by movement or by lying on the right side. Vomiting when present at this stage may be a pointer towards the disease. Many people label this stage as the stage of 'abdominal flu'.

The urine turns dark coloured and may not be much taken notice of. Some people may start with little itch at this stage. Slowly the patient passes into the jaundiced stage. But between the pre-jaundice and this phase there may be a short symptom free period of two to three days which very often gives the patient a false sense of relief.

Jaundice phase: As the patient passes into this stage now no doubts remain as to what is coming. Appearance of jaundice is heralded by the urine becoming more dark coloured and the stools becoming light coloured. This is the stage which generally comes by the 7th to 9th day of the initial start of infection. Jaundice now progresses and may reach its peak within 2 to 3 days. Within a few days the sense of well-being returns. The appetite returns and abdominal discomfort and vomiting cease. Patient may complain of itching but it does not last for longer period. Liver which is now well palpable is tender and constant pain may be complained of. The duration of icteric phase is about 2 to 3 weeks. Jaundice being at its peak within a week. Gradually the patient passes into the phase of recovery. The earliest thing which a patient notices is the improvement in the colour of urine which becomes light coloured and the stools which were clay coloured, their normal colour comes back. The jaundice also starts decreasing and sense of well-being appears. In a small percentage of people, jaundice phase becomes prolonged. Jaundice starts deepening and person complains of severe itching. This phase may last for few weeks but then recovery takes place which then is complete. This is the cholestatic phase (obstructive) and is often the cause of great anxiety to the patient and other family members.

Recovery or Convalescent phase: Generally recovery starts within a week or two after the onset of jaundice. There is a generalized sense of well-being with return of appetite which now is voracious. A smoker finds his urge to smoke coming back. The abdominal discomfort disappears and that constant ache over the lower part of right side of chest is no longer there as the inflammation of liver is now subsiding. But despite over all improvement, fall in bilirubin levels, return of normal colour of urine and stools, the patient still complains of generalized lassitude and fatiguability. This stage lasts from two to six weeks. But it is still prolonged in cases of hepatitis-B and non-A, non-B hepatitis. Total recovery is generally complete within a period of about 4 months.

On the whole a patient of hepatitis makes a complete recovery without any long-term ill effects.

But a minority of patients have a different course. A few patients of hepatitis may be seen with only mild form of the disease and often go unrecognized. On the other hand are those patients who show a very severe fulminating course. It may develop so rapidly that sometimes even jaundice may not be conspicuous. These patients have repeated vomiting, are confused and pass on to drowsiness and coma.

Development of hepatic coma is the most dreaded complication and is primarily seen mere in cases of hepatitis-B. The mortality is exceedingly high (about 80-90%) but those who survive recovery is complete. In a few cases as the patient of hepatitis is making good recovery from the acute phase there may be recrudescence of all the symptoms—fever, jaundice, malaise, etc. This is called relapse and is brought on by resorting to too early resumption of activity or the abuse of alcohol. Relapse form of hepatitis generally runs a mild course and recovery takes place. Some people may suffer from a number of relapses.

Another form to which a case of hepatitis may pass on is 'Subacute hepatitis' where the person instead of having complete recovery continues to have fluctuating levels of jaundice and low temperature. Some of such people progressively develop hepatic failure and death may occur. Those who survive pass on to post-hepatitis cirrhosis. This phase of liver involvement is very variable. A case of acute hepatitis passing on to subacute hepatitis goes into the picture of cirrhosis with the accompanying signs and symptoms, is easy to visualize. But there is this patient who apparently makes good recovery from acute hepatitis but returns after five years with fullfledged picture of cirrhosis. It only means that during the intervening period the changes have been taking place in the portal system and liver without apparently showing up.

After recovery from acute type-B hepatitis, a small percentage may become chronic carriers and these may develop chronic active hepatitis. This complication rarely, if ever occurs after hepatitis-A but may occur after non-A, non-B hepatitis.

If the patient of hepatitis fails to recover completely from jaundice, appetite and weight loss, fatigue and liver still remains enlarged with little tenderness, and even after a period of six—twelve months, the possibility of Chronic Active Hepatitis should be considered. Confirmation of the diagnosis is made by biochemical tests (elevated transaminases, bilirubin and alkaline phosphatase) and liver biopsy (bridging necrosis) findings in a case of protracted acute hepatitis.

Lastly there are certain group of people like doctors, nurses and educated elite who often have an insight into their disease and after complete recovery may start worrying about the possible ill effects of hepatitis. This phase is called 'Post Hepatitis Syndrome' and the whole picture is of anxiety, apprehension. Person may complain of easy fatiguability with failure to regain weight. Some may complain of tenderness in the liver area. All biochemical tests as well as liver biopsy in such people is normal and these people mainly require reassurance.

Diagnosis: Diagnosis of hepatitis is not difficult, provided one keeps one's eyes open during epidemics. Sporadic cases are detected if suspected. Once jaundice develops then there is no difficulty. Often cases of hepatitis have to be differentiated from the surgical causes of jaundice like gall stones, cancer, etc. But for this the treating physician is the best judge. In addition to the characteristic history, confirmation of the diagnosis shall be made by estimating bilirubin and transaminase levers. Absolute levels of the serum bilirubin have some prognostic value. Levels of 20 mg and above if persist, it indicates more serious disease. Similarly, enzyme levels may roughly tell us about liver cell damage. Very high levels (1000 IU or above) are not indicative of good prognosis. But as recovery takes place, the progressive decline takes place.

The presence of circulating HBsAG shall indicate type-B hepatitis. A diagnosis of type-A hepatitis shall be based primarily on negative serological testing for hepatitis-B markers.

Plain X-ray of the abdomen may be done to exclude gall stones. Liver biopsy is raraly undertaken and should preferably be not done in a case of jaundice unless the exigencies of the situation require it very essentially.

Prognosis: The overall prognosis in a case of hepatitis is good. Reported mortality in otherwise well fed people is about 1 to 2 per thousand people. Type-B hepatitis carries the highest mortality, since it is the commonest cause of fulminating hepatitis.

The prognosis depends on age, seneral health of the person and the promptness and adequacy with which the patient was treated during the pre-jaundice and jaundice phase.

The average young adult with uncomplicated disease has good prognosis and recovers completely within 6 weeks to three months.

Prognosis becomes poor in people who are anaemic, undernourished and are in poor health. This should not be difficult to appreciate as such people have got very poor resistance. Adequate treatment and bed rest definitely have a bearing on the further course of the disease. The risk of relapses is much more when bed rest during the acute stage of illness has not been strictly enforced.

Prevention: The basic approach in this common disease is prevention which is very important.

For hepatitis-A, control lies in maintaining, if not excellent, at least good levels of sanitation. Clean water supply must be ensured. Filtered drinking water is basic amenity in any civilized society. Factors like contamination of water supply by the public by ablutions must be stopped as contamination of water either by polluted water or sewage must be prevented.

During floods or breakdown in the water supply system water must be boilded for at least 15-20 minutes. Heavy chlorination of water is not adequate to destroy the viruses. Ultimate control shall be in safe disposal of faeces and proper control of insect vectors like mosquitoes, flies and cockroaches. Since the patient of hepatitis has already excreted the virus for sometime before he really developed jaundice so the virus has already been well disseminated in the community and at this stage isolation of the patient may not be of such use in preventing the further spread of disease.

Since the disease spreads by faecal contamination of food, water and milk, the patient must follow the elementary measures of hygiene like scrubbing hands thoroughly with clean soap and water after going to the toilet. Linen and other items of clothing of the patient should preferably be boiled and sterilized properly. Bed pans and excreta of the patient should be properly taken care of. There is no need to segregate the members of the household or the patient, though stress must be laid on maintaining adequate hygienic measures. In hospitals, barrier nursing is desirable. For close contacts who have not had previously hepatitis-A, further preventive measures may be taken in the use of immune serum globulin (ISG). It is effective in preventing or modifying the course of the disease and is also given to debilitated persons, young children and pregnant women during epidemics. Dose is 2-3 ml administered before or within one to two weeks of exposure. Hepatitis-A vaccine is also beneficial and has to be given to close contacts.

Hepatitis-B prevention means taking adequate precautions by health personnel working in laboratories, dialysis units, operating rooms and disposal departments of hospitals. All needles used by jaundiced patients must be handled properly. Those who handle human blood must take proper measures and must not soil their hands. The dangers from blood transfusions transmitting the virus can be, to a large extent, minimized by not using blood from professional donors. Similarly pooled blood must be avoided. If possible, all blood donors must be screened for Australian antigen.

All syringes and needles must not only be boiled for at least 10 minutes but also be autoclaved and then exposed to hot air for at least one hour. Preferably use disposable syringes.

Prophylaxis against hepatitis-B is recommended by the use of Hepatitis-B vaccine which is a non-infectious formalin inactivated subunit viral vaccine derived from surface antigen of hepatitis-B virus.

Dosage is 1 ml initially followed by 1 ml after one month and 3rd dose (booster) is 6 months after the first dose. It is to be given by intramuscular route.

This vaccination should be targeted to people who are at increased risk of infection and these are physicians and surgeons, dentists, nurses, paramedical staff and laboratory personnel handling blood, blood products and other patient specimens, selected group of patients like those in hemodialysis units and those patients who require frequent and large volumes of blood transfusions. Also in this category are blood bank and plama fractionation workers and also household and other intimate contacts of persons with persistent hepatitis-B antigenemia.

Management: No specific drugs are used for the treatment of hepatitis and whatever drugs are to be employed in a complicated case of hepatitis have to be done only under medical supervision. The basic principle of managing a case of hepatitis rests on two main principles:

1. Bed rest
2. Diet.

Bed Rest: There has been some controversy whether strict bed rest should be advised in a case of hepatitis or not. Whatever the critics of bed rest may say, the basic rule is that since the course of the disease may be unpredictable and an apparently innocuous or mild case may get into complications, it is wise to treat every case of hepatitis as a potential risk. Strict bed rest with only bathroom privileges must be enforced till:

1. the acute stage is over
2. the symptoms have disappeared
3. there is no jaundice
4. no tenderness or pain in liver area
5. serum bilirubin levels return to normal
6. enzymes (SGOT, SGPT) reach within normal range.

On an average, bed rest is advised for about 3 weeks. Once this acute stage subsides, little activity is allowed which is gradually increased till the patient resumes norms levels of active life.

If the patient initially is too ill, even bathroom facilities are to be provided by the bedside.

It is presumed that recumbency and bed rest induce enhancement of blood flow to the liver and in an inflammed liver, this coupled with very little activity hastens the recovery process. If symptoms of disease return, the patient must be immediately put to bed. Those patients who do no take adequate rest especially during acute phase run greater risk of developing serious complications of hepatitis. The convalescence should also be adequate so that recovery of liver takes properly. On an average, this period should be counted as double the period spent in bed during the acute phase. This may look very inconvenient to a person who is actively enagaged in his profession but ideally this is the minimum which patient must be askcd to follow in order to achieve proper health and well-being of his liver.

Diet: The basic principle of diet in hepatitis is to give nourishing preferably liquid diet in early stage comprising mainly of high carbohydrate and low fat contents.

In the acute stage when the patient is having loss or appetite and severe degree of nausea, it may not be possible to take solid foods. At this stage fruit-juices (orange, mosambi, sugarcane) carbonated drinks, lemonade, candy and sweet glucose biscuits may be given. Some patients may even require intravenous fluids to prevent dehydration and to gain calories. As vomiting and nausea subside, solid foods be introduced. Basic rule should be that this diet is palatable, nutritious, and easily digested. It should be divided into 5 to 6 small feeds rather than the usual 3 meals a day. The diet should provide 2500-3000 calories to the adult per day and out of this 350 to 400 g of carbohydrate should be comprising the main bulk of food content followed by 50-100 g of proteins and 50 g of fat.

High protein diet is not recommended in the presence of severe degree of jaundice, as there is danger of the person developing hepatic precoma. In fact at this stage proteins from the diet be eliminated or severely restricted. Scientifically there is no restriction to the use of fats, but an ill patient of hepatitis may find greasy food unappetizing or unappealing so the patient generally avoids such foods.

A diet high in energy and well balanced should preferably be employed. Well cooked and attractively served food will do more to restore the appetite.

Suitable food for persons suffering from hepatitis shall include boiled rice, fruits, jams, honey, syrup, chicken (tender) lean meat, boiled fish, eggs, finely sliced vegetables, potatoes, bread, custard, puddings, jelly, grapes, mangoes, lichies, chikoos, fruit juices, lemonade, etc.

Fried foods should be avoided. Heavy rich foods with excessive fats should also preferably be avoided. As recovery sets in, the diet should be brought to as normal levels as possible. An important precaution in any person suffering from hepatitis is to enforce complete prohibition of any alcoholic drink.

At the same time the alcoholic beverages must be forbidden to the patient who has recovered from hepatitis for at least six months to a year. This is very essential for the maintenance of normal health of the liver. In addition to the above, two principles additional supplements of vitamin B complex and vitamin C are given for whatever value they have. If not much benefiting these atleast assure the patient that something effective is being done. Moreover vitamins do act as somewhat protective for the liver and to some extent help the patient.

As the person moves on the road to recovery, general advice should be given to the patient about work, rest, diet and alcohol. The old principle of "prevention is better than cure" has definite place in reducing the morbidity and mortality of hepatitis.

Facts about Hepatitis

Viral hepatitis is of worldwide distribution and affects more than two million people. There are at least five viruses responsible for causing hepatitis, i.e., A, B, C, D, and E. No specific therapy is so far available against hepatitis, so it is important to employ preventive measures.

Hepatitis-A

It is a self-limiting infection and usually does not progress to chronic infection. The virus is excreted in faeces and spreads primarily by faecal oral route. Common source of infection is contaminated food or water. The infection is also acquired through close contact with infected individuals. It may be symptomatic in children and severity of infection is age-related with symptoms more severe in adults. Elderly stand the disease worst and recovery in them is often delayed. Symptoms may last from 6 weeks to 3 months and include nausea, vomiting, yellowness of eyes, malaise, fatigue, loss of appetite, etc.

Prevention of hepatitis-A is by adopting sensible practices of drinking pure water and eating healthy food.

Hepatitis-A vaccine has emerged as long term protection against the disease. A single dose (1 cc) followed by second dose after two weeks will give protection for a year and a booster dose after six months will afford protection for at least two decades.

Hepatitis-B

It has a more insidious onset and prolonged course than hepatitis-A. Of estimated 300 million carriers of Hepatitis-B virus (HBV) worldwide, 25-30% will die of hepatitis-induced liver damage. This virus is highly stable and resides in the host for a period of 15 years or more without showing any symptoms. Transmission is mainly by transfusion of infected blood and its products, use of contaminated instruments, syringes, needles, tattooing, acupuncture and unsafe sex. Vertical transmission from infected mother to child at the time of birth is another way.

This virus is mainly spread by parenteral route and is present in the blood during its long incubation period. Faeces of a patient of serum hepatitis unlike that of Hepatitis-A, are not infective. Hepatitis-B occurs at any age, has an insidious course and its incubation period ranges from six weeks to six months. Clinical features of the disease resemble any other form of hepatitis except that it follows a more serious course.

Prevention against Hepatitis-B means avoidance of professional donor's blood, screening of blood and its related products for surface antigen (HbSAg). All unnecessary pricks must be avoided.

Hepatitis-B vaccine gives effective immunization and is safe. It should be given to all persons at risk from hepatitis-B, persons coming in contact with blood or body fluids of patients, sexual contacts of HbSAg carriers.

These injections of vaccine at 0, 1, and six months are to be given intramuscularly in deltoid region, vaccine gives immunity in more than 95 per cent of people. For more rapid protection, third dose of vaccine can be given two months after the initial dose with a booster at 12 months. Vaccination is not recommended in pregnant women.

Non-A, Non-B, Hepatitis (Hepatitis-C)

This hepatitis is seen in drug abusers, homosexuals and after transfusions. In India 20 million people carry this blood borne virus. Clinical profile of the disease is just like that of Hepatitis-A and B, though less severe. Most cases develop chronic liver disease and even go to liver failure. Cancer of liver may develop in some cases.

Very little is known about prevention of Hepatitis-C. Hepatitis-C vaccine is not yet available.

Delta Hepatitis (Hepatitis-D)

It is caused by smallest known virus which rides piggy back of Hepatitis-B virus. It is mainly transmitted by parenteral route, in drug addicts and after transfusion. Delta Hepatitis is uncommon but produces severe form of Hepatitis with a more severe course. There is no separate vaccine against it, though infection by this virus can be prevented by giving Hepatitis-B vaccine in susceptible individuals.

Hepatitis-E

It is due to water borne infection and is closer to hepatitis-A virus. It spreads through food and water. The clinical picture is acute, all ages are effected but more so in young adults. The course of the disease may be prolonged and severity waxing and waning for many months.

Prevention of Hepatitis-E is similar to that of Hepatitis-A, i.e., improved sanitation and provision of purified water supply.

CIRRHOSIS OF LIVER 5

Cirrhosis of the liver is widely prevalent all over the world and its incidence varies from country to country, depending on the dietary habits, alcohol intake, social and religious customs of people. It is not possible to assess the number of people suffering from it in the population at large, since a large number of people may not have any symptoms for a long time. It is a disease which follows a relentless course and unless adequate steps are taken in time to halt the onslaught of the disease, it rapidly progresses and ultimately leads to premature death.

Annual death rates from cirrhosis of the liver have been in the range of 2 to 20 per 100,000 populations. These figures would be variable depending on the causative factor. One would appreciate that alcohol which is responsible for the production of alcoholic cirrhosis shall definitely monitor the fatality rates in the population depending on its consumption—higher the alcohol abuse in society, higher the morbidity and mortality of cirrhosis of liver.

Let us look at the disease itself. Cirrhosis has been derived from the Greek work 'KIRRHOS' meaning 'TAWNY'. This is so because if one looks at the livers of people dying of cirrhosis, one shall find that there are multiple nodules projecting from the liver surface and are of fawn or yellowish-russet colour bordering on the greenish. The main characteristics of a cirrhotic liver is extensive disorganization of the hepatic lobular architecture. All parts of the liver are involved. There is diffuse liver cell death with hepatocellular necrosis, and formation of scar tissue with regenerating cell masses.

The causes of liver cirrhosis shall vary in different parts of the world. In more than 50 per cent of the cases, no factor is responsible and this type is called "Cryptogenic". Next in importance is alcoholic cirrhosis which is probably one of the commonest causes of cirrhosis in the Western society. In North and South America, Europe and United Kingdom three quarters or more of portal cirrhosis patients are associated with alcoholism. In our country and other countries in the tropics, malnutrition probably accounts for a great majority of sufferers followed by that which is the end result of hepatitis.

In addition to the above factors responsible in the production of cirrhosis of liver there are other uncommon causes like prolonged cholestasis, toxins, drugs, disturbed immunity and metabolic factors. Basically in cirrhosis there is significant loss of liver cells followed by collapse and fibrosis of the reticulin network. The whole liver is distorted and there are areas where liver cells are trying to regenerate and form nodules. Thus we have death of liver cells and there is overall scarring of the liver. Regeneration of the liver takes place secondarily. This picture invariably is present in all persons with cirrhosis irrespective of the underlying cause. The end result is the same in all varieties. As the cirrhotic picture progresses, the presence of fibrosis leads to distortion of the vasculature (intrahepatic vascular system) in the liver and this contributes to the development of rise of pressure in the portal system (portal hypertension). But what are the factors which contribute to the development of liver cirrhosis. Let us look at some of them.

Hepatitis: Some people who suffer from hepatitis develop cirrhosis later in life. Depending on the severity of the disease process, some may develop at a very early stage. However, studies on soldiers who had hepatitis in epidemics during World War II and in the Korean War have shown not any increased risk of developing cirrhosis.

Some of the studies have shown that people suffering from hepatitis (Type-B, non-A, non-B) with extensive liver damage can progress rapidly to cirrhosis (post-necrotic) and similar is the case with those who suffer from chronic active hepatitis. It is not always essential to get history suggestive of hepatitis in large number of sufferers of cirrhosis. In fact cirrhotics either do not remember or even mention any history of having suffered from hepatitis. But those who do give the history the percentage is very less and only ranges from 3 to 17 people out of 100 cases of hepatitis. This has been the experience in most of the epidemics of hepatitis all over the world. But there is a discordant note. Following the epidemics of hepatitis that occured in 1933 and 1943 in Denmark, an increased number of cirrhosis of liver was observed amongst women in the period between 1944-1948.

A causal relationship between hepatitis and subsequent development of cirrhosis cannot be ignored. Moreover, the fact that a person does not give history suggestive of hepatitis does not exclude it as mild forms of hepatitis might be either ignored or missed by the person.

Malnutrition: It is common to see patients with cirrhosis liver presenting with malnutrition. Whether poor nutrition per se produces cirrhosis of liver is controversial. The fact that dietary deficiency in animals produces picture resembling cirrhosis led to a probable role of nutrition in the causation of cirrhosis in human beings.

The hastened development of cirrhosis in alcoholics is due to a number of factors and out of them poor dietary nutrition does have some role to play. Interestingly, fatty liver produced in alcoholics in early stages is also produced in persons who suffer from severe degree of protein malnutrition (kwashiorkor) but there is no evidence that such people are at increased risk of developing cirrhosis in later life. Protein malnutrition is especially common in undeveloped countries. There is evidence of its effects on the various organs of the body and liver is no exception. It also suffers with other organs.

The role of nutrition in the causation of cirrhosis is disputed. The only indication of cirrhosis induced by malnutrition was observed in epidemic form in China during Japanese occupation. It is presumed that since hepatitis is on the increase in many parts of the world, it along with malnutrition may be responsible for cirrhosis which is being attributed to malnutrition. In fact a number of factors like toxins, chronic ingestion of contaminated food, parasitic infestations and alcohol may complicate the picture in a malnourished person. Malnutrition will have an indirect role to play in such type of people. It either makes the liver more sensitive to injury or accelerates or exacerbates the underlying liver pathology leading to cirrhosis.

The role of nutrition can be summed up as follows. Deficient diets such as are eaten by people in undeveloped countries have an indirect effect on the liver. They predispose it to injury by various agents like toxins, parasites and viruses, etc.

Cryptogenic (*Idiopathic*): It means of obscure or unknown origin and that is what some of the people suffering from cirrhosis of liver may be having. It has been said that in the West at least half the persons suffering from cirrhosis have no cause or underlying disease to explain why they have got it. These people do not have any history suggestive of having suffered from hepatitis or been jaundiced. Even the history of excessive alcohol abuse is not there. Some of these do give history suggestive of alcohol but it is in moderate amount and not sufficient enough to produce liver injury resulting into the picture of cirrhosis.

Interestingly cryptogenic cirrhosis occurs more in English people compared to Americans. One estimate puts approximately 50 per cent of English cirrhotics to be cryptogenic, while amongst the Americans there is only an incidence of 10% who belong to this category. There is one interesting comment by an English physician who, when asked about the paradox of this type of cirrhosis, quipped, "An average Englishman cannot afford enough amount of alcohol which should be of sufficient quantity to produce alcoholic cirrhosis." This is not totally a correct picture but it only tries to bring the point that alcohol is not the commonest cause of cirrhosis amongst Britishers and that is why people think it to be cryptogenic.

To look at the Liver of such cirrhotics is not in any way different from that due to other causes. It has got nodules (macronodular) but the characteristic picture of alcoholic cirrhosis is missing. There is a lurking belief that all so-called cases of cryptogenic cirrhosis had probably an inapparent hepatitis earlier on or some unknown cause like susceptibility to environment,

Malnutrition or toxins which might be playing a part in the background.

Alcohol: The role of the alcohol in the causation of cirrhosis of liver has never been underestimated. Alcoholics have a high incidence of cirrhosis, though it may take almost ten years for an alcoholic who takes about half a pint of gin, beer or whisky a day to reach the stage of cirrhosis. Studies from various centers in the world have shown that alcoholic cirrhosis occurs seven times more common in alcoholics than in non-drinkers and this association is closely related to the amount of alcohol consumed per day. Though association of alcohol and cirrhosis is well established, yet it is again said that associated factors like nutrition, infections and toxins also play a role and shall accelerate the whole process. Once cirrhosis develops, it pursues a relentless course and even withdrawal of alcohol has a limited beneficial effect, since the process is a continuous one, though the survival may be prolonged. Often a view has been put that it is not the alcohol per se which causes cirrhosis but there is some other factor in the beverage which is the real culprit. Evidence has been brought forward to show that in the United States, cirrhosis occurs predominantly in whiskey drinkers, in France, Italy and

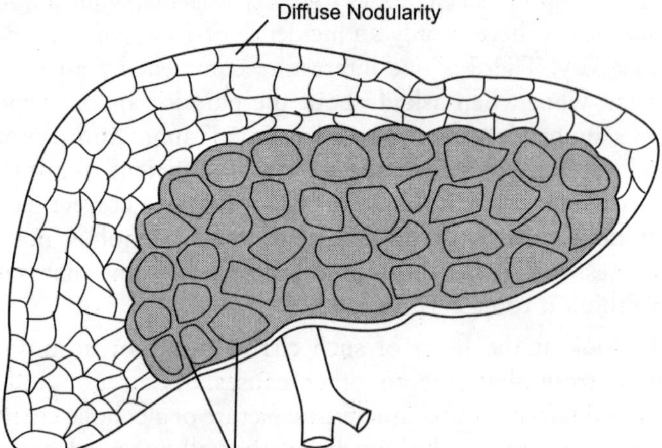

Liver: As it looks in Cirrhosis

Germany in wine drinkers and in Australia in beer drinkers. The only common factor in all such cases is alcohol. Strange are the habits of people in some other places. In France cirrhosis is associated with the consumption of red and not white wine, while in Spain port wine and not sherry have been blamed to be the real culprit.

But some of these factors have not been well substantiated. All available evidence points to the fact that it is amount of alcohol consumed rather than the type of beverage that shall affect the person's chances of developing cirrhosis.

The earliest lesion of alcoholic liver disease is fatty infiltration which is rapidly reversible and is not to be considered in any way an irreversible process and on that a pre-cirrhotic one. But if alcohol consumption is not stopped at this stage and no remedial measures taken the person is going to pass into the stage of alcoholic hepatitis. This is a serious condition and at this stage even when alcohol is stopped some degree of liver damage is going to persist which may further worsen if the person again gets addicted to booze. The end result of alcoholic abuse is cirrhosis which accounts for 75% of cases of cirrhosis amongst Americans and 25-30% of all cases of cirrhosis amongst the English people.

In addition to disturbances in the architecture of the liver and excessive reticulin formation with fibrosis there is presence of Mallory Hyaline Bodies in the liver which represent the ultimate of alcoholic insult to the liver. It is a paradox to say that occasional drinker does not develop liver damage, though even some chronic heavy drinkers also have no signs of any deleterious effects of alcohol on their liver. An occasional drinker gets only a transient liver injury because it is the continued drinking of hard liquors over a number of years which produces the damage. Why progressive liver damage occurs only in certain people is due to the genetic linked association. Immunological hyperreactivity may be responsible for the progressive destruction of liver cells. That is why some people who have stopped taking alcohol and are now taking good diet they still develop cirrhosis. It is important that one must heed the early signs of alcoholic liver injury and take remedial measures.

Miscellaneous: We have discussed the common factors which account for vast majority of cirrhotics. But then there are still a number of people where some obscure factors might be operative. Thus prolonged cholestasis (both intra and extra hepatic) where there is obstruction to the biliary tract due to some compression (congenital or acquired) is subsequently going to lead to the development of cirrhosis. Small quantities of insecticides like DDT if ingested over long periods might cause cirrhosis. Similarly, exposure to small amounts of industrial poisons like trichlorethylene is going to result in liver damage provided the exposure has been over a period of 20-30 years. One would appreciate that it is difficult to have people who have been exposed to the same chemicals for such long periods and then the history may not be very helpful.

Warning has come over prolonged use of drugs like Methotreate (a widely used drug for leukemias, etc.) Isoniazid (antitubercular), methyl dopa (antihypertensive). It has been found that incidence of cirrhosis was higher when small frequent doses of these drugs were employed over long periods rather than large intermittent doses. Factor of disturbed immunity is also known to play its role in this multifaceted disease. A host of other factors like familial, ethnic, racial and genetic predisposition combined with disturbed immunological response are going to play their role in association with nutrition, infection, alcohol, etc. in the production of cirrhosis. It cannot be oversimplified to say that one factor alone does not cause cirrhosis. Other factors shall contribute to progress of the disease in some way or the other.

Picture of Cirrhotic Liver: Liver in cirrhosis has a very typical appearance and can hardly be ignored. It is generally enlarged and varies in weight from 600 to 4,000 g. It is on the whole larger in alcoholics. People who have had cirrhosis of long duration, the liver is shrunken, small in size and is studded with fine uniform nodules.

More than one and a half century back Laennec described the cirrhotic liver. This description is so perfect that one cannot help quoting it, "The liver reduced to a third of its ordinary size was, so to say, hidden in the region occupied: its external surface lightly mamellated and wrinkled, showed a greenish yellow tint: indented it seems entirely composed of a multitude of small grains, round or ovoid in form, the size of which varied from that of millet seed to that of hemp seed. These grains easy to separate one from the other, showed between them no place in which one could still distinguish any remnant of liver tissue itself; their colour was fawn or a yellowish russet, bordering on greenish, their tissue rather moist, opaque, was flabby to the touch rather than soft and on pressing the grains between the fingers, one could not mash but a small portion; the rest gave to the touch the sensation of a piece of soft leather." Large livers are seen in cases of alcoholic cirrhosis as majority of them die in early stages because of either liver failures or intercurrent infections. The liver at this stage is pale, since it is fat-filled. As scarring develops the liver turns grey or green.

Liver does not have smooth appearance. It is studded with uniform nodules varying in size. There may be granularity when nodules are small but when they become large, there are areas of broad depressed scars separated by scar tissue and large granules. In fact the normal lobular pattern of liver is destroyed which now is divided and sub-divided by bands of connective tissue forming what is called Pseudolobules.

In sum total a cirrhotic liver whatever its cause, is just a remnant of its normal self.

What is the appearance of a cirrhotic? A person who has had his/her liver damaged is hardly going to present a picture of good health. A patient of cirrhosis may present in three forms. Firstly are those who come and seek help for their symptoms and signs. These are the ones who have a fully developed picture of cirrhosis and constitute more than 60 per cent of the total group. Second group falls into the latent group where the person is not ill and the disease is detected coincidentally during evaluation for a routine medical check up or when he is being examined for some other diseases. Third group is that in which the diagnosis is made only at post mortem. This also constitutes about 30-40 per cent of the group. Such people have a low profile of the disease and often remain undetected during their lifetime.

The earliest complaint of a cirrhotic is loss of appetite and the person feels that he is not in his normal spirits. He gets easily fatigued, complains of generalized weakness and weight loss. If the person is an alcoholic, he often gets further compulsion to take more alcohol, since to his mind alcohol shall be the panacea for his state of ill health, thus further accentuating the liver damage. Some of these people after a heavy bout of alcohol may land up in the hospital with acute liver injury.

Gradually loss of appetite is followed by nausea, abdominal pain and vomiting. Liver cell failure which has started manifesting itself with these complaints becomes progressive and the general health of the person starts failing. A low grade fever indicating liver cell necrosis and gram negative bacteraemia develops. Soon jaundice may appear. It colours the skin and urine assumes a dark appearance. The very fact that jaundice has appeared means extensive liver cell destruction. At this stage the liver has lost capacity for regeneration and indicates a serious course of events.

Fluid (ascites) appears in the abdomen which assumes a distended appearance and is protuberant. Before the person really shows up with ascites there is abdominal distension and flatulent dyspepsia. Gradually swelling also appears over the legs and feet but fluid in the abdomen always overshadows the fluid in the legs.

The general appearance of a cirrhotic is very characteristic. He has got a bloated appearance with a typical facies in the form of sunken eyes, pinched nose and hollow cheeks. A typical 'family' likeness which is not difficult to appreciate. The skin is pale, waxy and often is pigmented. There are fine vessels at various parts of the body (spider naevi) which look like a tiny spider and in fact are dilated vessels present over cheek, shoulders, breast area, chest and abdomen. These have also been called 'paper money skin' and are indicative of a hormonal imbalance due to liver dysfunction. There may be bleeding from the skin at various places. The hands show reddish pigmentation (palmar erythema), a spotty redness on the hands eminences and in the pulps of the fingers. The nails assume a typical white appearance and may rarely be clubbed.

As a result of endocrinal disturbances, body hair is often diminished and a male person shows female distribution of hair. In some, hair may disappear completely and the person may have a boyish appearance with less recourse to shave. Some people loose hair from the rest of the body and it may not be uncommon to find a cirrhotic with a clean hairless chest.

All said and done, hardly any system in human body escapes the effects of cirrhosis. One of the earliest signs may be the appearance of enlarged parotid glands (situated on the face) which are painless and soft. The size of the gland regresses as the liver functions improve.

Cirrhotics have inflammation of gastric mucosa (gastritis) and the incidence of peptic ulcer is on the higher side in them. A cirrhotic has a full bounding pulse. The limbs are warm. Sweating is usually absent in severe form of cirrhosis. Axillary hair both in men and women are scanty. Pubic hair in men assumes feminine characteristics. A very distressing feature in men is the development of feminization or female characteristics which is primarily due to inability of liver to metabolize the female hormone (Oestrogen). Men develop prominent breasts (gynaecomastia) which is a distressing sign. There is atrophy of testicles. The male patient complains of decreased sex urge (libido), impotence and suffers from sterility. In females, menstrual irregularities occur. There may be complete cessation of menses (amenorrhoea). The breast and genital organs show atrophy. Some of the sexual dysfunctions both in men and women may improve with improvement in hepatic functions.

As said earlier, abdomen is distended. Liver is often enlarged, firm or hard and irregular. In later stages it becomes shrunken and may not be palpable. Spleen is enlarged in great majority of people. Veins over the abdominal wall may be dilated and prominent.

In advanced forms of liver cirrhosis the person may develop neurological signs in the form of apathy, slowness and brevity of response with disturbed sleep rhythm. Personality changes in the form of irritability, lack of interest in family and impairment of intellectual functions leading to gross confusion develop.

Gradually speech becomes slurred, the voice monotonous. With further deterioration, signs of hepatic failure with progressive weakness of limbs, disturbed consciousness, tremors, flaps and coma may develop.

Development of coma in hepatic cirrhosis is a very grave sign, since it carries high mortality. Even in the best of hands and with all facilities available, death rate in hepatic failure goes up to 90 per cent.

Hepatic failure in cirrhosis might be precipitated by injudicious use of opiates and sedatives, anaesthesia, infections, electrolyte disturbances and bleed in the food pipe or stomach. Some of the cirrhotics may present with severe vomiting of blood which occurs due to rupture of blood vessels in the food pipe or stomach (oesophageal or gastric varices) and indicates rise of pressure in portal system (portal hypertension). Such people are also liable to have excessive bleed from piles which, though less life-threatening, may be extremely persistent. So if one looks at the total spectrum of the disease in a cirrhotic individual one would appreciate that it is a silent killer which spreads its tentacles to all the systems of the body.

Diagnosis and investigations: A great deal depends on how true a person is in telling about his diet, extent of alcohol abuse to his doctor. Earlier the suspicion, better is the prognosis, since withdrawal of alcohol in any person goes long way in reversing the process.

Besides all the features of cirrhosis enumerated earlier, the diagnosis can be made by number of investigations. Liver function tests may show raised bilirubin levels. Albumin content of blood is diminished but gamma globulins are raised. Serum alkaline phosphatase is raised and so are the enzymes. Varices in the oesophagus are detected by barium meal study and further confirmed by endoscopy.

The exact degree of liver damage can only be assessed by doing a liver biopsy when a small piece of liver is taken by means of needle (Vim Silverman's or Meghini type) and examined under the microscope. This shall show the characteristic abnormalities suggestive of cirrhosis. Needle biopsy of the liver is an invasive procedure and has got its own hazards.

There have been further advances in the diagnostic procedures in the evolution of non-invasive techniques. These include ultrasonography, computerized tomography and radio isotopic scans. Splenoportovenography is another investigation which is a safe procedure and requires the use of dye to visualize portal venous system.

Diagnosis and the type of investigations shall to a large extent be judged by the treating physician, since it is all an individualist approach, and every person requires individual planning.

Management: The specific ways of managing a cirrhotic shall not be delineated here, since these require the guidance of a competent physician. We shall only discuss the general measures. Basically depending on the underlying cause the management varies but the basic rule of provision of adequate nourishing diet supplemented by vitamins especially of vitamin B complex group cannot be minimized.

Most of the cirrhotics have loss of appetite, so ensure that that diet is appetizing, wholesome and nutritive. If anaemia is present it has to be corrected by the use of haematinics. If alcohol is the offending agent, it is very essential to take the patient away from it. For this the will power on the part of the person as well as cooperation of friends and family members is very essential to wean the person away from this pernicious habit. There is an erroneous belief amongst certain people, including doctors that an alcoholic liver is a result not so much of drinking 'gin before dinner' as 'gin instead of dinner'. This means that a proper diet rich in nutritions taken after drinks can look after the health of the liver. It is an erroneous belief and must be removed from the mind of the alcoholic. The very fact that a liver starts showing signs of early liver dysfunction, it is a warning signal to completely abstain from alcohol.

Some of the cirrhotics have a feeling of ill sorts that they call as 'liverish'. This is to be treated symptomatically and shall improve as liver functions improve. One must be very cautious about the use of certain drugs like analgesics, tranquilizers and sleeping tablets, etc. in cirrhotics as such people react very badly to them and their liver dysfunction may be further worsened.

For those who develop portal hypertension, portal caval shunt surgery may have to be undertaken. Bleeding from varices can be controlled by sclerotherapy (injecting of drug in the veins) and if required in some cases by resection. Medical measures in the form of drugs like pitressin and beta blockers like propranolol are also being employed to lower portal pressure.

Prognosis in a case of cirrhosis shall depend on a number of factors. It has been rightly said that cirrhosis need not be a progressive disease and with adequate measures the downhill progress may be halted.

Alcoholic cirrhosis responds better if detected early and if complete abstinence from alcohol is followed. Presence of jaundice is a bad sign, since it indicates extensive liver dysfunction. A large size liver means that the cirrhosis is in early stages, while the shrunken liver indicates an advanced stage.

Resistant to treatment, appearance of complications like bleeding varices, hepatic pre-coma and coma, gross alterations of biochemical tests and extensive liver damage (as shown by liver biopsy) all indicate bad prognostic signs.

To conclude cirrhosis of liver is a multifaceted disease which is preventable in some and not in others. Those who have got a known cause, they can prevent the onslaught of the disease process provided they cooperate with their doctor.

Liver Transplantation

During the last few decades advances have been made in transplantation of liver. This is a very specialized procedure which requires high degree of precision and the set up of specialized units. Here expertise of surgeon performing liver transplant as well as well-trained nursing and para-medical staff is very important.

Potential candidates for liver transplantation are children and adults who suffer from severe irreversible liver disease for which alternative medical or surgical treatments have been exhausted.

In children biliary atresia is the most common condition requiring a transplant. Here there is progressive distortion of bile ducts in the liver and this leads to cirrhosis of liver and liver failure. Metabolic disorders which are genetically transmitted and are associated with progressive liver failure both in children and young adults, are another field which require a liver transplant. The commonest indicator for liver transplantation is case of end stage liver disease where all other measures (Drugs, exchange transfusion, plasmaphresis, haemodialysis and charcoal haemoperfusion, etc.) have earlier failed or been exhausted. Transplantation in cases of carcinoma liver is generally not undertaken as the recurrence of malignancy is high.

Patients with life-threatening systemic diseases, infections, pre-existing cardiac or respiratory diseases and malignancies are not good candidates for liver transplant. Even in patients with alcohol related liver disease, results of transplant are rather disappointing.

Transplant may be total or partial. In the post-operative period most patients succumb to infections. Immunosuppressive therapy has to be given and may be continued life long. Rejection of graft occurs in majority of patients one to six weeks after surgery. Chronic rejection of liver transplant is relatively rare.

Prognosis in all cases of liver transplant is guarded. Children fare slightly better than adults. Children who survive initial three post-operative months, one year survival rates are 96 per cent as compared to 89 per cent in adults. Five year survival is seen in more than 50 per cent of cases. Quality of life after surgery is not bad and one has to guard against possible chances of infection, etc. Some women who underwent transplantation and received immunosuppressive therapy have also conceived and carried the pregnancy to full term without any demonstrable ill-effects to the child.

LIVER AND INFECTIONS 6

Whenever the body is exposed to severe degree of infection its major organs bear greater part of its ill-effects manifested either by anatomical damage or functional dysfunction. In this category, liver is no exception.

Liver is involved in various cases of infections. These may be as varied as pyogenic, amoebiasis, tuberculosis, typhoid, malaria, syphilis, relapsing fevers, kala azar, hydatid disease, liver flukes and roundworms, etc.

There was a time when pyogenic liver abscess secondary to severe degree of infection or pyaemia present in gastrointestinal tract or in the adjacent organs was considered a life-threatening problem with almost hundred per cent mortality. Those were the times when there were difficulties in making diagnosis and localizing abscesses. But we have travelled a long time since then and in the antibiotic era, the management and treatment of such cases has improved. Still there may be cases who may have either single or multiple abscesses. Depending on whether the abscess is single or multiple and whether management has been on medical or surgical means the prognosis will vary.

The most significant and important affection of the liver is amoebic. Since amoebiasis is endemic in our country and probably more than 90 per cent of our population suffers from it because of the insanitary and unhygienic conditions, it is no wonder that liver is going to be involved in some way or the other.

Entamoeba histolytica is protozoal parasite which has its abode in the large intestines and has invasive properties—invading both the tissues and the intestines. The organism may exist in two forms—the vegetative (highly infective form) and a more quiescent or dormant form — the cysts. Most people may be chronic passers of cysts for a long time. But the cyst has the uncanny property of surviving in most unfavorable circumstances in the environment. When swallowed by the individual either through food or by fingers contaminated with it, it passes unaffected through stomach and intestines and gets converted into the vegetative form in the colon.

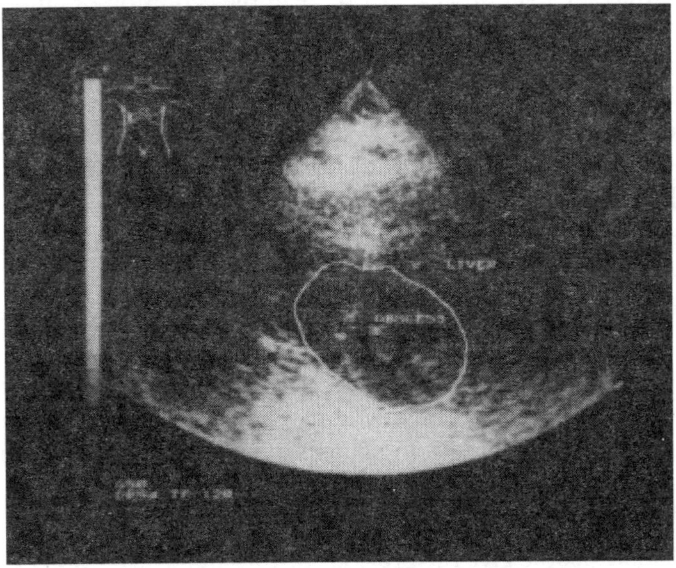

Ultrasound of Abdomen showing Liver Abscess

From there the amoeba invade the liver like parachutes dropping in the battlefield. These amoeba reach the liver via the portal veins and start multiplying there, initiating an inflammatory process. The liver has got a moth eaten appearance with areas of necrotic tissue surrounded by areas of congestion. The overall appearance of liver is that of diffuse inflammation with areas of necrosis containing degenerated liver cells.

If the invasion of the liver by amoebic infection is overwhelming, the end result is formation of an abscess. Most of the times the liver abscess is formed as a result of fusion of a number of small areas of necrosis. Generally there is a single large abscess present in the right lobe of the liver. More than one abscess may also be present. An abscess in the liver is surrounded by fibrous lining with shaggy necrotic tissue. In the center is the brownish red pus often called as Anchovy (since it resembles this type of sauce) with necrotic debris of liver tissue and E. histolytica also lying there. Though it is called 'pus' yet in fact it contains no pus but only degenerated cells and liver tissue.

Amoebic liver abscess is a stage in the evolution of amoebic infection of the liver and sometimes there may be hardly much differentiation between the stage of amoebic hepatitis and abscess. This is governed by the virulence of amoeba and the degree of resistance present in that person. A debilitated or weak individual who suffers from amoebic infection is more likely to fall prey to it than a comparatively well fed person.

As said earlier, right side of liver has more predilection for involvement. Eighty per cent of liver abscesses are present in right lobe of liver, 10 per cent in left and the rest may be present in both.

The onset of the disease process is slow. Usually, a patient of amoebic hepatitis presents with occasional fever and sweating. These may be the only complaints for a number of weeks. Then the person may start complaining of loss of appetite, ill-health and pain in the liver area or in the upper part of abdomen.

Some people give the previous history of loose motions with or without blood or mucus while in some there may be no such history available. Very often the patients in our country ignore these occasional complaints of abdominal discomfort or bowel irregularity.

On a rough estimate an untreated case of intestinal amoebiasis develops involvement of liver within 3 months. Some people may take even years before they show any signs of liver involvement. The infrequent occurrence or delay in such people is probably due to the treatment for amoebiasis which they might have been taking. Again it happens that some people do not get their intestinal disease treated adequately. Moreover they are constantly being exposed to repeated infections so that a stage of poor health may come when liver gets involved.

As liver involvement progresses, instead of hepatitis, the abscess forms. Now there is progressive deterioration of health, loss of energy, lassitude, signs of toxaemia in the form of fever, flatulent dyspepsia and may be bowel irregularity. The patient has a peculiar sallowness of the skin like earthy tan, it is so typical that once seen, there is no mistake about it. There is a dull aching pain in the liver area which becomes sharp and severe. Sometimes the pain is referred to the shoulder. This pain is more marked at night and even movements of any kind may accentuate the pain.

The liver is enlarged, tender and painful. Pressing on the lower part of chest on the right side may evoke pain. If the abscess in the liver is lying superficially it may start pointing towards the outside. Rapid expansion of the abscess will again produce severe degree of pain.

Liver abscess, if not treated in time, may rupture either into the abdomen or into the lungs. When it ruptures into the lungs, the person may expectorate blood into sputum. Very often the whole pus from liver abscess has been expectorated out. Though it looks like blood in the sputum, a careful examination will show that it is not really blood but rather anchovy pus.

Once a suspicion of amoebic involvement of the liver has been aroused, confirmation can be made by investigations. Blood count shows a moderate increase with rise in polymorph cells. Serological tests (complement fixation and haemagglutination inhibition tests) are helpful. Screening of diaphragm for movements will show it to be restricted. X-ray of the chest will show elevation of the dome of the diaphragm on right side and a peculiar 'HUMPING' indicating an abscess pointing towards the lungs. Further confirmation of the lesion can be done by aspirating the abscess or by scinti scanning. Stools may or may not show entamoeba histolytica cysts.

The most common complication of amoebic liver abscess is its rupture either into the lungs, pleura, pericardium or abdomen. Secondary infection may supervene when the patient becomes more severely ill. Jaundice may be present in a case of amoebic liver abscess either in later stages or when it is very big. Treatment of amoebic infection of the liver is done under medical supervision. Drugs which are effective against intestinal as well as tissue invasion are desirable. Very effective therapy in the form of dehydroemetine, tinidazole, metrondiazole (flagyl) choroquine and furamide are employed. The choice of drug and its duration is to be judged by the physician. Alcohol should not be taken by a patient of amoebic infection of liver for obvious reasons.

If abscess is present and is pointing towards the surface or even deep seated but not responding to treatment, pus should be aspirated.

Prognosis in a case of amoebic liver abscess is good provided the diagnosis is made early and the proper treatment instituted. Poor health, presence of complications like secondary infection or rupture shall worsen the condition. But overall results are good. After recovery the person should be advised to take antiamoebic course of drugs at regular intervals for residual infection which might be lurking in the intestines. Similarly adequate precautions for protection against reinfection from amoebiasis must also be taken.

Tuberculosis involves liver like any other generalized infection but there is no peculiarity about it. Some of the drugs used for treatment of tuberculosis like isoniazid, rifampicin, etc. may cause liver damage. Again because people being exposed to receive repeated injections and their general resistance being poor, they are more liable to contract hepatitis-B.

Other infections also involve liver to some degree but shall not interest a lay reader.. Round worm infection is very common in our country but rarely these worms invade the liver and biliary passages, even causing fatal results. Sometimes the worm enters the common bile duct and produces obstruction with resultant jaundice and cholangitis. Very rarely the worm may burrow itself in the liver even perforating or rupturing it with very disastrous results.

An infection of the liver which cannot be ignored is Hydatid disease of the liver. It is widely prevalent all over the world and has existed since times immemorial as when the man acquired close proximity with its best friend—the dog.

It is caused by swallowing the ova of the echinococcus or hydatid worm which lives in dogs. Dogs act as definitive hosts, while man, sheep and other cattle may act as intermediate hosts.

The dog gets infected by eating viscera of sheep which is infected with hydatid. These enter the dog's intestines and there develop into the adult worms. The ova are shed into the intestines and thus infect the canine faeces which are now a very potent source of infection. These infected faeces now contaminate the grass or farmlands and from there are ingested by sheeps, pigs or even camels. Man gets infection by playing with the dog whose almost every part starting from skin, paws to muzzle has been contaminated and fingers of a man are the real culprits. Even licking by a loving pet is going to convey the infection. Further infection is going to result from the use of infected vegetables, contaminated water, salads, etc. which have not been washed properly with clean water or been cooked inadequately.

Once the eggs are swallowed, their outer covering is dissolved by gastric juices and the liberated ovum now burrows through the wall of the stomach or intestines and reaches liver via portal vein route. Once it reaches liver, generally its further passage is arrested. It is caught in the liver mesh (sinusoids) and now forms a small cyst with outer covering. After a time some buds project from the cyst wall (endocyst) and develop into daughter cysts. These are just like mother cysts and soon become independent entities. Cyst contains a clear fluid in which there are hooklets or hydatid heads.

Liver is involved in more than 75 per cent of the hydatid disease cases and it is only a small percentage of victims where the ova pass through the liver and are lodged in other organs of the body like lungs, spleen, brain, etc.

Proper disposal of waste products from slaughterhouses, maintenance of adequate sanitation and taking precautions while handling pets as well as using vegetables, etc. well cleaned and washed up are the measures essential for prevention of hydatid disease. No wonder in places where dogs have unrestricted access to infected faeces and offal, the incidence of hydatid disease is going to be alarming. Except for some developed countries of the West like Britain and U.S.A., almost all countries of the world including Australia, Newzeland, Africa, South America, Europe, Greece, Middle East, Canada, India, Pakistan, Turkey, etc. have a very high incidence of the disease.

A hydatid cyst in the liver may produce no problems for a pretty long time and the person remains in good health till it may be detected accidentally or even after death.

It is the increasing size of the cyst which gives a feeling of fullness and weight in the liver area. Sometimes an accidental blow received over the abdomen may rupture the cyst and person may collapse. Very often the sufferer may notice a small rounded swelling in the liver area and it may start pushing forward. It may rupture into the abdomen, into the bile ducts or even into the lungs. Once rupture occurs, secondary bacterial infection occurs and now the picture is not a silent one but that of an abscess with fever, toxaemia, etc.

Since hydatid cyst contains fluid, which has foreign material, when this cyst ruptures the patient may experience a severe allergic (anaphylactic) reaction. Rarely the hydatid cyst may become quiescent. Its gets calcified and looks as if it has now become inactive.

Suspicion about hydatid in liver should arise when a round cystic swelling is felt in a reasonably healthy person without any obvious complaints. Diagnosis can be confirmed by complement fixation and haemagglutination tests. Casoni test is not very reliable. X-ray of the abdomen may show a calcified cyst. Further help is obtained by hepatic scanning and ultrasound.

Management of hydatid disease of liver is both preventive and therapeutic. Prevention is very important. Dogs should not be allowed to feed on raw offal, since it is a very potent and dangerous source of infection.

Dogs should not be petted or allowed to lick the person till one ensures adequate hygienic measures like cleaning of hands, etc. by antiseptic lotions. The owner of pet must ensure that a veterinarian handles the general health of the animal regularly by the use of proper deworming agents in the dog so that source of infection could be eradicated. At the same time dogs excreta must also be disposed of properly. Since there is danger of rupture of the cysts, it is advisable to remove the hydatids surgically, though complete removal of the cysts is virtually impossible.

Medically mebendazole for a period of 3 weeks to one month is considered an effective line of treatment.

In sum total hydatid disease may remain asymptomatic for a pretty long time in any person without producing any ill-effects but once complications occur, the overall morbidity increases.

Thus one would appreciate that liver is a victim to number of infections and the effect on it can be variable, depending on the cause of infection and its subsequent sequelae.

LIVER IN INFANCY AND CHILDHOOD

7

We have talked in detail about the afflictions of the liver in adult but the question may arise whether liver in infants and children is going to behave in a manner different than that in adults?

There is no doubt that liver has some peculiar differences in children and infants and there are certain interesting properties which require further elucidation. At birth liver is a tiny organ weighing about 120 to 150 g constituting about 4 per cent of the total body weight. With the development of child there is going to be proportionate development in liver size as well. It assumes twice its weight of birth at the age of one year and to thrice at the age of 2-3 years. This increase in weight occurs rapidly and thus is now six times the original weight by the age of 9 and almost 10 times at puberty. Though the increase in weight of liver is adequate with age, yet it does not go parallel with the overall body development and the increase is less than that of the body as a whole, being merely 2 per cent of the body's total weight.

The topography of the liver in infants is different from that of adults. The left lobe of liver is relatively larger in newborns but with progressive development of the child this changes as well with the result that at the age of eighteen months the liver of the child now resembles exactly like that of adult liver in its anatomical characters. In fact the basic character of the liver has already been established by the age of one year.

What about the functional working of the liver? There is no doubt that liver has undergone rapid changes leading towards maturation in its perinatal life and much depends on the infants capacity to deal with its environment. There is evidence to show that the functional capacity of the liver is not fully developed at birth and this understandably is going to be more pronounced in premature or immature infants.

The most important and common manifestation of liver involvement in infants is the appearance of jaundice which appears by the second or third day after birth and lasts for one to two weeks. It is transient and harmless and that is why it is called physiological jaundice. Apparently the appearance of jaundice in the infants becomes a source of anxiety to the parents. But this requires reassurance about the innocuous nature of the jaundice.

The possible reasons for this jaundice is the delay in conjugation of bilirubin, since the new born's liver is burdened with an excessive load of the unconjugated form of bilirubin and there is delay in clearing it by the inefficient transport system of the neonates. This defect is soon corrected and the liver assumes its normal functioning and that is the reason why this jaundice starts disappearing by the 5th to 7th day after birth and the infant is completely free from it by the 2nd week. But things are going to be more difficult in premature infants where the whole mechanism of liver suffers from more serious functional insufficiency. The jaundice in such infants appears early, lasts longer and may assume more serious profile. When jaundice in these children reaches abnormal proportions, the child may develop rather graver complications (kernicterus). In this condition also called bilirubin encephalopathy, the infant is restless, does not take feeds because of loss of sucking reflex. Some children are lethargic, febrile and may develop a stiff neck and generalized rigidity. Depending on the severity, even death may result in these infants. Some even die in a period of few hours while more than 60-70 per cent succumb to it within seven days of the onset of the jaundice. Those who survive are left with mental defects.

Another interesting type of jaundice which does not appear in every infant is called breast milk jaundice, which is seen in only 1 to 2 per cent of babies fed on breast milk and is said to be due to the presence of an undefined substance in the breast milk which interferes with the bilirubin conjugation. The jaundice appears on the sixth or eighth day and may last from two weeks to eight weeks after the delivery. Interestingly when breast-feeding is stopped, the jaundice also disappears. But if in this period breast-feeding is resumed, the jaundice reappears. This jaundice, which is seen only in a few infants, is mild, non-injurious and does not harm the infant in any way.

In contrast to the above varieties of jaundice, we have more serious forms of it which result due to either increased haemolysis or destruction of red blood cells. These are the results of antigens in the foetal blood cells which have initiated the development of antibodies in the mother which lead to destruction of foetal red blood cells. The result is the appearance of jaundice in the first 24 hours of life and is the result of Rh. incompatibility. This is what happens to the offsprings of Rh+ve and Rh–ve parents. Isoimmunization develops—the first child of such parents generally escapes the ill-effects and it is the first pregnancy which has sensitized the mother's blood to such a degree that it now provokes destruction (haemolysis) in the next pregnancies. The degree of jaundice in such children is variable. In some it is mild while in others it may be of really pathological levels and produce extensive damage to the infant. The affected infants are pale, jaundiced and are swollen (oedematous) with severe degree of anaemia. Some infants may be still born. Suspicion of Rh. Isoimmunization is anticipated when mother's blood has been tested for Rh. typing during check up.

This type of entity carries bad prognosis. In majority of places, prevention is being achieved by the administration of potent anti-D gamma globulin to such mothers after each delivery or abortion or miscarriage so that they destroy fetal Rh+ve red cells that enter the mother's circulation at the time of pregnancy. In such children where severe degree of haemolysis is present, exchange transfusions are helpful and have saved numerous lives. Next in importance to Rh. haemolytic disease is the one which results due to ABO or other rarer blood groups incompatibility. There are also cases of increased bilirubin soon after birth which is due to some enzyme deficiency (glucose 6-PD) which is further worsened by the use of drugs like antimalarials, salicylates or sulphonamides passed into the mother's milk and thus produce jaundice in the infant.

Rare condition associated with decreased bilirubin uptake, storage and conjugation is the condition called Criggler-Najjar syndrome which is associated with the deficiency of an enzyme. It is a serious condition associated with severe jaundice and presents a very serious prognosis. If above is a serious condition then we have mild forms of neonatal jaundice like Gilbert's disease where jaundice is mild and may not be noticed even till adult life. Jaundice in an infant may be due to other diverse causes. If there is infection round about the umbilicus, it may spread along the umbilical vessels to the liver. Even systemic infection of severe degree is going to produce it. Jaundice appears all of a sudden in a child who has been perfectly healthy earlier on. Depending on the acuteness of the condition the child may be more seriously ill. Outcome of the condition depends on how promptly the condition is diagnosed and treatment instituted. Very small infants and undernourished ones carry high mortality.

But let us not ignore the fact that even hepatitis can occur in infants which is due to hepatitis-B. It develops in babies of those mothers who had suffered from the acute disease during the later part of pregnancy. Some of the mothers are asymptomatic and infect the infant either through the mother's blood during delivery or later on when the infant is being nursed. The baby may have a mild form of hepatitis or even avery severe form. This hepatitis in those infants who survive usually results in chronic hepatitis and ultimately may go to a fullfledged picture of cirrhosis. Still there may be infants where though picture like hepatitis is present, yet the cause has not been established. This is the idiopathic type of hepatitis which may be running in the family.

When jaundice appears after the first week of life, then the picture is that of obstructive type. It is characterized by marked rise in levels of bilirubin (both direct and indirect) and not only is prolonged but is progressive. Commonest cause of this type is congenital obliteration of the bile ducts. There may be biliary atresia which very often cannot be corrected by any surgical procedure. Jaundice is deep and progressive, imparting an olive green icteric tinge to the skin. Itching is marked. Saliva and tears of the child are bile stained. The stools are clay coloured and urine is dark coloured. For several months the infant may remain in good state of health but gradually weight loss occurs. The child now becomes lethargic and less alert. Severe degree of diarrhoea may also occur. Intercurrent infections may kill such children. Majority of such infants do not live beyond two years of age.

Of the rare causes of jaundice in infants, mention may be made of some infections in the mother which are responsible for the production of jaundice in the new born. These include syphilis, rubella, herpes simplex and viral infections. Still rarer causes will be glycogen storage disease, galactosemia and alpha-1-antitrypain deficiency.

But as the child grows up, another set of causes of jaundice may be operative. Of this group the important are hereditary haemolytic anemia where there are defects in the red blood corpuscles. This shall comprise cases of hereditary spherocytosis, thalassemia (mediterranean anaemia) and sickle cell anaemia. These children present with anaemia, mild jaundice, dark coloured urine and faeces. The basic defect is in the red blood cells whose normal life span of 120 days is reduced to as low as 15 to 20 days. Jaundice may be increased because of periodical haemolytic crisis. Once severe jaundice appears, the chances of early remission disappear. Though haemolytic anaemias have a different factor responsible, yet as jaundice forms an important part of their presentation so one must keep these in view in children having severe anemia, jaundice, retarded growth and chronic ulceration over the legs.

Now let us look at the spectrum of various diseases affecting liver in childhood. Hepatitis either due to type A or B is in no way different than that in adults except for the fact that in children below the age of five, hepatitis presents with little or no jaundice. Once the jaundice is severe the child may rapidly assume a downhill course and may go into hepatic failure. Relapses in children are frequent as compared to adults. Prognosis and survival from hepatitis in children is directly proportional to the nutritional state of the child.

Cirrhosis of the liver in children again has got varied etiology. It may be cryptogenic or follow an attack of viral hepatitis.

In India we have got a variety of cirrhosis which is a distinct entity prevalent in our country. As a report from Indian Medical Council says, "Infantile cirrhosis of the liver is a disease peculiar to India affecting infants and young children, with a tendency to run in families. It is characterized in the early stages by enlargement of the liver which is felt to be hard and usually also of the spleen with ascites (swelling of the abdomen) and jaundice superimposed in the later stages. Its onset is insidious with vague symptomatology, course variable but generally rather slow and usually the termination is fatal. Its etiology is unknown.

Indian childhood cirrhosis has certain peculiar characters. It runs in families who are basically pure vegetarian. Children of Bania Aggarwal group and Hindu Brahmins are more prone to suffer from it, though Mohammedan and Christian children are also affected but their percentage is not very high. Children affected belong to 1-3 years age group and it has got a familial incidence. Both sexes are equally affected.

Various theories have been put forward from time to time to explain why it runs in families. Genetic factor along with a common environmental factor is said to play an important role. This is well illustrated by the example of a man who had two wives and children by one wife were healthy whereas those by the other wife, all breast fed, died of infantile cirrhosis.

The onset of the disease is usually slow and insidious. The early symptoms are rather vague. Parents may notice the child to be dull and morose with little appetite. The child has liking for more sweets and carbohydrate foods rather than the proteins in the diet. The skin looses its glossy appearance and jaundice may be seen.

Often by the time disease is suspected the liver is considerably enlarged. Child may be irritable or peevish. An irregular fever is invariably present. At this stage there is no ascites. Further progression of the disease results in the liver shrinking in size. Jaundice is deep and there is full-fledged picture of cirrhosis, fluid in the abdomen, swelling of legs with generalized emaciation.

Child is ill and irritable, spleen is palpable. The overall picture of the child is of severe hepatic dysfunction, characterized by loss of weight, generalized emaciation with protuberant abdomen, swelling of legs and feet with jaundice present in varying degrees. Once liver failure supervenes the prognosis is poor.

Treatment of Indian childhood cirrhosis is unsatisfactory. Basic approach should be to improve the diet patterns of families where the entity runs. Proper antenatal care of the mother, infants feeding practices and adequate attention to the nutrition in the early period of life will give the child some protection. Institution of measures to provide good nutritious diet with substantial proportion of proteins in a balanced diet should provide at least some protection to the child from the clutches of this relentless disease. There may be some hope in it, since the etiology of childhood cirrhosis still remains a mystery and is anybody's guess. Hereditary, nutrition, infection, metabolic and immune factors may have some role to play.

Of the other diseases affecting liver in childhood probably the pattern is the same as in adults. Amoebic hepatitis and liver abscess have the same mode of presentation and clinical course. Again one is more likely to see amoebic infection of the liver in slightly older children. An occasionally palpable liver should not frighten the parents of a child, since a number of benign conditions may enlarge the liver and make it palpable.

Tumour of the liver in infants and children are very rare. Moreover, the suspicion, diagnosis and management of most of the liver ailments in infants and children has to be under medical supervision. It is very important to understand this, since children are rather fragile and delicate and any mistake made in this regard may lead to irreparable damage and even fatal results.

So, handle a child with liver problems with care.

HOW TO MAINTAIN A HEALTHY LIVER

8

A number of years back the famous magazine 'Punch' put a question to its readers. "When is life worth the living?" The most interesting answer given was, "It all depends on the liver."

Often the word going round the party circles of elites is, "How is your liver today?" Is it because the body's most versatile organ is controlling the person's moods and behaviour patterns since it is said that man's attitude is to a large extent being controlled by the health of his liver.

A bad liver in the common man's Jargon has been said to make that person peevish as a wasp and on the other hand, a healthy and kicking liver makes that man cheerful and sweet. Very often in olden times people used to talk about 'Liverishness'. It used to be a form of term applied to that feeling of uneasiness which develops in people who over-eat and consume large quantities of carbohydrates, but without adequate quantities of proteins in the diets. Such people often feel out of sorts, are irritable, depressed and complain of a feeling of general rundown, headache and even drowsiness. There is excessive flatulence and often a felling of bloating in the abdomen. It is considered that liver in such people is inactive and is not probably activated to meet the demands of excessive carbohydrates in the diet. Often there is worsening of the liverish feeling by the alcohol abuse. Some people may complain of discomfort in the liver area.

This brings home to us the significance of the use of a well balanced diet. Palate tickling foods and richly seasoned dishes entail an excessive strain on the liver, since they take long time to digest. If this habit is repeated ad lib the liver may have to do more work and at the same time it is being deprived of proteins and vitamins which are equally essential for the maintenance of its well-being.

A liver for keeping its health requires adequate quantities of carbohydrates, proteins and fats in the diet.

Carbohydrates (350-400 gm), proteins (100 g) and fats (50 g) per day constituting 3,000 calories of diet for an average individual is what constitutes the basic requirements of a normal person. This food, to do its duty, must supply enough energy, nutrition and be palatable and easily digestible.

Plenty of fruits, milk, lean meats, rice, poultry, etc. shall constitute important supplements to the diet of any person. Sweets, pastries and very rich greasy and fried foods have to be avoided.

A person who feels liverish must see to it that he avoids dry fruits, nuts, gravies, soups and rich food. These should be substituted by fresh vegetables, salads, fruits, fruit juices like orange, mosambi, etc. Of the fruits, grapes, oranges, mangoes, water melons, jack fruits, pineapple are good. Of the non-vegetarian food, chicken, fish and lean meats are easily digestible. Eggs and milk should also form a part of one's daily menu. In other words a well balanced, nutritious diet shall go a long way in maintaining the health of liver. Lack of proteins in diet despite its being rich shall produce a fatty liver.

Tea, coffee, cocoa, etc. can be taken in moderation. Coconut water is a good nourishing drink.

We have talked about giving a nutritive diet for maintaining the health of liver in any individual. But take the case of a person who has an already damaged liver. In such people though carbohydrates have to be given in adequate amounts but proteins have to be restricted since proteins given in large amounts may further precipitate liver damage as a result of excessive production of ammonia and nitrogenous products in the intestines. Well compensated cases of cirrhosis will require adequate quantities of first class proteins for the regeneration of liver tissue.

Malnutrition especially of proteins gives rise to liver damage with the result that it may shrink (in starvation) or enlarge (protein malnutrition). Pre-existing malnutrition may make the liver more prone to injury by toxic and infective agents. At one end of scale under-nutrition produces changes in the liver, while at the other end obesity also produces a fatty infiltration of the liver. This may look a paradox but then it is explained on the fact that diet of the obese people is mostly composed of either carbohydrate or fats and is woefully deficient in proteins. So the best way to manage liver of an overweight or obese person is to make attempts to reduce weight but without compromising on the proportion of first class proteins in diet.

A word may be mentioned here about herbal teas and bush teas which are often taken by people for medicinal purposes. These concoctions are injurious to liver and so should be avoided.

Alcohol is anathema to the maintenance of good health of the liver. The old notion of taking alcoholic drinks with food and not that of alcohol instead of food does not hold true now. Alcoholic injury to liver cannot be prevented by the use of high protein or nutritious food. So prolonged use of gin, beer, whiskey, sherry or any alcoholic drink should be prohibited for the sake of maintaining a healthy liver.

Whenever a person consumes alcohol a little injury to the liver is produced and if further exposure to the beverage is done, the damage will be perpetuated.

An occasional peg may not harm the person. But the problem arises when alcoholic spirits overpower the individual's will power and he becomes an addict. There is a very slender thread between a social drinker and an addict.

To minimize injury to the liver the minimum any person can do is not to consume alcoholic drink within the next 24 hours so that the liver is able to tide over the harmful effects of alcohol in that period.

Where liver damage has occurred in any way and it has become vulnerable, even small quantities of alcohol are dangerous, and alcohol must be avoided. Exposure to alcohol in a case who has suffered from cirrhosis is nothing short of throwing that man into the lion's den. Similarly any person who has had hepatitis must avoid alcohol during the next 6 months to 1 year. Avoidance of alcohol is a pro qua non for any person who wants to maintain his/her liver. An occasional alcoholic drink is not taboo but one must watch against the occasional dip and an addiction.

A very important consideration about maintaining health of liver is the effect of drugs on the liver. Drugs when taken orally are mainly metabolised in the liver. This occurs through a method of enzyme inducers. The full utilization of a drug depends on the health of the liver and its cells (hepatocytes). Thus in a damaged liver the utilisation of drug will be affected.

Injury to liver by the drugs may be mediated by certain metabolites which combine to deactivate the toxic substance or by means of an immune reaction. Interestingly the first mechanism is dose related to the amount of drug consumed while the second mechanism is unrelated to the dose of drug.

A number of drugs are being used in day to day practice. Some are being prescribed by the doctors, while some are being taken by the people of their own. One physician wrote "it is not difficult to compile a list of more than hundred drugs which cause liver damage." Further on, it was remarked that it is probably an understatement. The wise policy is to regard any drug as a potential liver poison.

All types of liver damage or injury is produced by the use of certain drugs. It must not be out of place to mention here that those with an already damaged liver, howsoever mild the damage might be, run the added risk of getting drug toxicity much earlier than an absolutely healthy liver. The two common sorts of liver injury produced as a result of drugs shall be either hepatitis or cholestasis. Some drugs may produce even severe hepatic necrosis. This has resulted from the use of heavy metals (gold, mercury), large doses of paracetamol and intravenous tetracycline especially in pregnancy. Hepatic necrosis has been worsened by certain fungal and plant toxins. This state develops rapidly and in a very short time the person goes into hepatic failure within a period of 24 to 48 hours.

Some drugs are associated with the production of a picture resembling hepatitis and it includes a list of drugs ranging from anti-tubercular drugs (isoniazid, pyrazinamide, rifampicin, ethambutol), barbiturates, antirheumatic drugs (phenylbutazone, indomethacin) and drugs used for gout (probenacid, allopurinol) to appetite suppressants. Drugs which produce cholestasis include chlorpromazine (Largactil) calmpose, anti-depressants, anti-diabetic drugs (tolbutamide chlorpropamide, phenformin) anti-thyroid drugs, diuretics (chlorthiazide, frusemide). Anti-histamines to anabolic hormones including male sex hormone.

Let us look at some of the drugs which are very much in common practice.

Toxicity with tetracyclines is increased in the presence of protein malnutrition. It is significant that heavy doses of the drug when given intravenously is more likely to produce harmful effects. Paracetamol taken for longer periods is likely to produce liver damage which may be in the form of toxic injury to the liver or chronic active hepatitis. This ill effect of drug on the liver results more in those who have already a damaged liver or suffer from malnutrition. Same picture of liver injury may result due to chronic use of salicylates.

Hypersensitivity type of drug reactions occur with isoniazid with further acceleration if this drug is combined with another anti-tubercular drug called Rifampicin.

A very mild form of liver injury may occur due to the use of anti-hypertensive drugs (methyl dopa). Liver injury also occurs due to the use of sulphanomides, erythromycin, nitrofurantoin (urinary antiseptic), anticonvulsants (dilantin) and anti-inflammatory agents. These effects generally take about 3-4 weeks to show up and are more marked in people who are chronic users of these drugs.

A very significant consideration is about the possible ill effects on liver after the use of oral contraceptives (The Pill). This is related to the content of sex hormones in the drug. Attempts have been made to reduce the content of active hormone in the drug to further lessen this side effect. So it is always a safe policy to warn women who are on the pill about the possible harmful effects of the drug on liver.

To look at the problem of harmful effects of drugs on the liver, one must consider that liver with an already damaged base, in the presence of malnutrition and women during pregnancy run added risk of potentiating the liver injury. Apparently for the proper utilisation of drugs and maintenance of liver health it is very essential to be conservative about the use of certain drugs especially if the liver is damaged.

To summarise one must appreciate that liver—the vital organ of the body—can be kept healthy if:

1. Nutrition of the individual is adequate and there is no evidence of the person suffering from protein malnutrition. Diet must be well balanced with an adequate proportion of first class proteins derived both from vegetable and animal sources.
2. Alcohol consumption must be limited and one must be moderate in one's habits. For those who have a damaged liver, alcohol use is taboo and even a single drop should be considered nothing but poison.
3. One must avoid the use of herbal; preparations since a majority of them are known to produce liver injury.
4. Indiscriminate use of drugs and self-medication must be stopped. You never know what danger is lurking in that tablet which you are popping in.

If your liver is healthy, you will feel cheerful and more healthy. So keep it healthy. It does not cost much, since a few principles of sane living followed diligently shall go a long way in maintaining your liver and ultimately prolong the quality and span of your life.

9 GALL BLADDER, GALL STONES AND FATTY DYSPEPSIA

Gall bladder is an important organ of the human body and has very close relationship with the smooth functioning of the liver. Situated on the visceral surface of the liver along the line which separates the right lobe of the liver from the left, is a thin bluish pear shaped organ what we call as gall bladder. It consists of a fundus, a body and a thin neck tapering to form the cystic duct which joins the common hepatic duct to form the common bile duct and finally terminates into the second part of duodenum (upper part of small intestines).

The major function of the gall bladder is to concentrate and store bile which in turn is secreted by the liver and delivered into the duodenum at appropriate time to assist in the process of digestion. This process is further governed by hormonal and nervous factors. Any factor which interferes with the normal functioning of the gall bladder shall produce both organic and functional disorders of the biliary system.

Cholecystitis means inflammation of the gall bladder. It is one of the commonest ailments of the organ and in more than 90 per cent of the cases is associated with gall stones. It is only 10 per cent of the minority group where there are no stones.

Cholecystitis may come on either in acute form or repeated attacks of mild to severe form of the disease process produces the condition meriting the diagnosis of chronic cholecystitis. Acute inflammation of the gall bladder is brought on by obstruction in the cystic duct caused either by an impacted stone, stricture or any structure pressing from outside. This is further worsened by the superimposed bacterial infection. The gall bladder becomes distended, greyish red in colour with a lustreless surface. Depending on the severity and chronicity of the attack it may become distended (acute attack) or thickened and contracted if there have been repeated attacks. Sometimes in very severe cases gangrene of the gall bladder may develop.

Persons who suffer from attacks of cholecystitis are generally obese, above the age of 40 and females who have had repeated pregnancies. But it does not mean that thin persons, men or those in younger age are immune from the disease. They also suffer but their number is less.

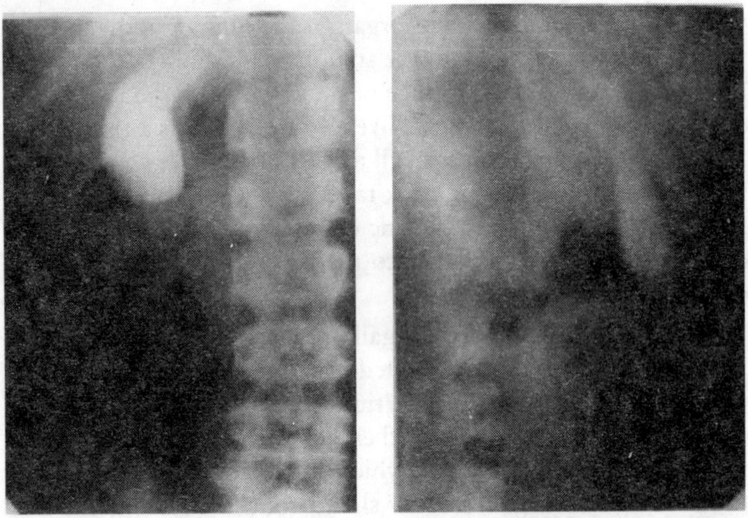

(a) **(b)**

Cholecystogram showing normally filled gall bladder (a) and same after fatty meal (b).

It indicates a normally functioning gall bladder.

There is generally an acute attack of pain coming on either at night or in the early hours of morning. It is present commonly in the upper part of abdomen on right side and is colicky in nature and very commonly pain goes to the shoulder and back. Often the attack is brought on by late night parties or heavy meals or fatty foods. Pain does not subside completely, though it reaches its peak levels in between. There is nausea and vomiting. Patient lies curled up in bed and is in agony because of the pain.

Jaundice may appear if there is obstruction in the common bile duct.

Diagnosis of this condition is made by the physician in great majority of patients on clinical examination. Confirmation is done by further investigations. Blood count is raised. Plain X-ray film of the abdomen may show gall stone. Intravenous cholangiography or isotopic scanning is of value. Ultrasound or CT scanning is the investigation of choice, the diagnostic accuracy being more than 80 per cent.

Patients with acute cholecystitis are treated on conservative lines, which includes bed rest, liquid diet, antibiotics and pain relieving drugs. Surgical intervention is not done in the acute stage until and unless there are dire indications for it like gangrene of the gall bladder. As a rule, surgery for acute cholecystitis is undertaken at a later stage when the acute process has subsided.

Repeated attacks of inflammation whether mild or severe are ultimately going to convert the gall bladder into a thickened fibrosed structure which is unable to concentrate bile. The whole process may come on insidiously. The gall bladder is small, contracted, pearly while to look at and contains bile which is turbid and the gall stones (which have a very close association with chronic cholecystitis) may be seen lying loosely embedded in the wall or the meshes of the fibrosed network round the wall of the organ. There are debris present all over.

A sufferer from this condition often complains of chronic dyspepsia, indigestion and vague abdominal discomfort of no specific character. There is flatulence, a sense of fullness and excessive belching. Abdominal distension or epigastric discomfort may be brought about by either a large or fatty meal. There is dull mild sort of pain in the upper part of abdomen on right side. Nausea is common but vomiting may not be there.

The significant sign of chronic cholecystitis is tenderness in the gall bladder area. Confirmation is made by plain X-ray film of the abdomen, cholecystography, ERCP, cholangiography and ultrasonography. There are generally gall stones present and the gall bladder shows poor functioning.

Patients of chronic cholecystitis are treated both medically and surgically.

As most of such people are fat, reduction in weight is very desirable. Patient should be advised to take fat-free food. The treatment of choice is surgical until and unless there are pressing reasons for not undertaking it like poor health of the patient or presence of some complicating illnesses.

In addition to the above two presentations of cholecystitis often associated with gall stones, there may be a very small percentage of patients where picture is like that of cholecystitis but no stones can be demonstrated. This condition is frequently diagnosed on the basis of flatulent dyspepsia and a gall bladder which is non-functioning. Causes of this type of cholecystitis can be trauma to the abdominal wall, infection (typhoid, generalised bacterial infection) surgical operations, diabetes and use of certain drugs like steroids.

But the most frequent ailment involving gall bladder is gall stone disease which is a major health problem in many parts of the world. An estimated 20 million Americans have gall stones and one million develop them each year. American-Indians particularly of PIMA Arizona have probably the highest incidence of gall stones and these are very common amongst people in Western countries like United States, England, France, Germany, Sweden, etc. The MASI tribesmen have very low incidence of gall stones. More industrialization and urbanization towards Western dietary habits are going to be major factors in the increased incidence of cholesterol gall stones as compared to pigment stones in the Third World countries. Environment, social customs and dietary factor play an important role. Japanese population in Hawaii has an higher incidence of gall stones as compared to their kinsmen in the main land.

Gall stones occur in varying degree in all races and populations, though the incidence varies from country to country and people to people. The Framingham survey has shown that 8 per cent of the population in the 30 to 60 years age group had symptoms of gall bladder disease. Gall stones are equally common in our country, though it may be difficult to really define the exact incidence, since no such studies are available but the factor of increased dietary intake of fats, sedentary habits of the people are going to play an important role, since gall stones have gone side by side with the growth of civilization. More affluence, urbanization and increased consumption of rich diets by the people means an higher incidence of the disease.

Gall stones are of three types—cholesterol stones, pigment stones and the rare forms of calcium carbonate stones. Very often mixed forms of stones are present. The composition of stones varies from time to time. You may have one type of gall stone at one time and the other one at other time. Cholesterol stones are large, yellowish and round as well as the more common multiple faceted 'mixed' stones which contain at least 70 per cent cholesterol.

Pigment stones are small, irregular, mulberry like in shape, friable and are very dark or black-brown in colour. They represent about 25 per cent of the stones. Pigment stones are very common in the tropics whereas cholesterol stones are common in the Western countries. Interestingly in urban Japan the composition of gall stones is changing from the pigment type to the cholesterol type for very obvious reasons.

Calcium carbonate stone is mere chalky white paste and is often bile stained. It often co-exists with other types of gall stones.

What are the factors which predispose to stone formation? These are variable and range from age, sex, genetics, diet, obesity to some known and some unknown factors. There is very common amphorism. 'Fat, forty, female, and full of flatus'. This is often quoted and misquoted in favour of gall stones but it is not always true.

10 per cent of the population of all age groups in United States suffers from gall stones and this prevalence is doubled in those over the age of 40. There is no doubt that the incidence of gall stones increases with advancing age. But gall stones can occur at any age, though the overall incidence remains definitely in the age group of 40-50 years.

Genetics may be playing an important part, since certain families are stone formers. Whether it is genetics or environmental plus social factors which play its part in such people is difficult to say. But on an average 20 to 30 per cent of patients with gall bladder disease have some other member of the family also suffering from it.

Gall stones are more common in women as compared to men, the incidence being almost double before the age of 40 but with the onset of menopause the incidence in both sexes is almost the same.

Pregnancy is an important factor in the genesis of gall stones. Females with multiple pregnancies have higher incidence. Pregnancy induces a change in the physiology of the biliary system: there is increased concentration of bile which becomes more viscid, cholesterol levels are elevated and emptying of gall bladder is impaired especially during the last months of pregnancy. The increased concentration of bile and cholesterol, aided by stasis favours formation of gall stones. In women during the post-menopausal period who are on oestrogen containing drugs and those on oral contraceptives, the incidence of gall stones increases implicating the role of sex hormones.

Obesity also plays a significant role. Gall stones are more common amongst obese and this is probably related to increased cholesterol synthesis. Certain diseases are associated with a greater likelihood of gall stones. Pigment gall stones are more common with disease in which haemolysis is frequent. These are six to seven fold far common in patients with cirrhosis including primary biliary cirrhosis.

People who are on cholesterol lowering diets such as those high on unsaturated fats and vegetable fats but low in saturated fats run an increased risk of gall stones. Similarly, cholesterol lowering drugs such as clofibrate commonly used in cases of heart disease are also associated with an increased incidence of gall stones.

Factors like diabetes, obesity and hypercholesterolemic states (high levels of cholesterol in blood) have an important association in the formation of stones. But why stones form is not really known. A number of factors have been incriminated. An important factor is the increased concentration of bile which is further governed by infection in the gall bladder, stasis and alterations in the composition of the diet consumed. But what changes the normal composition of bile to make it more concentrated (lithogenic)? Liver has often been blamed for it.

Cholesterol stones can form when the secretion of cholesterol into the bile increases or bile salt secretion is diminished. Both factors play complimentary role to each other. The factor of diet is equally important. A rich diet is definitely going to determine the lilthogenecity of bile.

Thus though gall bladder is the main site of gall stones, yet one cannot ignore the role of host of other organs ranging from liver, intestines to metabolic and hormonal influences. Gall stones may remain silent and produce no complaints. Often there is heaviness in the right upper abdomen made worse by jolting. There is dyspepsia which is either continuous or present intermittently. Some who suffer from gall bladder dyspepsia complain of short attacks of pain occurring at any time of the day or night with or without any obvious cause. Surprisingly these attacks may be worsened by a long railway journey, a drive on a bad road or violent exercise or some trauma over the abdomen. The intervals at which such attacks occur are variable. Occasionally, there may be long periods of freedom from the ailment.

Typically, symptoms from gall stones are associated with either an acute attack of cholecystitis or when the stone starts passing into the cystic duct. There is acute pain in the upper abdomen or in the area of gall bladder. There is restlessness, nausea, profuse sweating and slight rise of temperature. Jaundice appears as the stone reaches the common bile duct, but it is often intermittent.

In the period between the attacks, the patient may appear quite well, though a slight degree of jaundice or some residual pain in the gall bladder area may be present. If the stone remains impacted for a long time sooner or later cholangitis is likely to develop.

There is an interesting phenomenon called 'the disappearing gall stones'. Often there are reports of gall stones which were demonstrated unequivocally on X-ray films and have disappeared without the intervention of the surgeon. Very small gall stones pass through the normal passages during the attack of gall bladder colic and may be passed out, resulting in natural cure. A large gall stone may pass through a fistula (abnormal passage) between the gall bladder and intestines (duodenum or colon) into the bowel. These fistulae generally develop over long periods without much symptoms and result due to adhesions produced due to chronic inflammation of the gall bladder. Rarely gall stones may be expelled spontaneously even without the presence of a fistula. Gall stones that appear during pregnancy or in the period following delivery of the child have been known to dissolve and thus disappear.

Diagnosis of gall stones is part radiology and to some extent clinical assessment. One can suspect the disease from the history. Only about 10 per cent of the gall stones are radio-opaque. Pure cholesterol stones are never visible on the X-ray but when lime salts are present, they show a characteristic ring shadow. Most of the times, gall stones are multiple and faceted.

Cholecystography (oral and intravenous) is essential for assessing gall bladder function as well as to demonstrate the stones. Further help can be sought from ultrasound or CT scanning. ERCP is equally helpful in demonstrating the stones in the gall bladder and in the bile ducts. Question arises as to what is going to happen if the gall stones are left as such?

A majority of the gall stones may remain silent and thus asymptomatic and painless. Often controversy has arisen whether these stones are really innocent. Many believe that 'innocent' is a misnomer for these stones and rather a myth. Even if there are no symptoms it is a better practice to remove them rather than suffer from complications later on.

When gall stones produce symptoms there are no two views. These cases have to be treated. The desire of some people to avoid surgery has resulted in the evolution of drug chenodeoxycholic acid used for the dissolution of gall stones.

Small radiolucent gall stones in a functioning gall bladder can be expected to dissolve in 60 per cent of the cases.

The drug acts by improving cholesterol solubility by reducing liver synthesis and biliary secretion of cholesterol. Dose is approximately 1g daily and it may have to be given over a period of 6 months to 2 years. Small stones may show signs of dissolution at about six months, while larger stones take longer time, may be two years.

Initially when put on this drug, patient may show improvement in his symptoms. Diarrhoea is a very common side effect of the drug. A fair percentage of patients after dissolution of gall stones may show recurrence after a year also.

But do we advise this type of treatment in every case? Basically this line of treatment is advised in very elderly patients who are poor surgical risk or in cases where there are contraindications to surgery because of other complicating diseases like cardiac or renal pathology.

Cases with non-functioning of the gall bladder as shown in cholecystography, large stones, multiple and calcified stones, obese and those with complications are the people where medical treatment is not going to be of any help.

The surgical approach in all such cases in cholecystectomy where the offending gall bladder with gall stones is removed.

Diet and gall bladder disease: A close relationship between diet and gall stones formation has been incriminated. People who consume excessive quantities of fats, meat and cholesterol containing food have higher incidence of gall stones. Lack of dietary fibre in diet, use of processed foods and excessive consumption of foods containing fats and cholesterol have a definite bearing on the role of these factors in the causation of gall stones. Primitive people living on simple diets have almost insignificant incidence of gall stones, thereby suggesting that diet does have a role in the production of gall stones, though the evidence is mostly indirect.

Studies carried out by Prof. Yudkin have shown that all species of animals are adopted anatomically, physiologically and bio-chemically to a particular part of diet and it probably takes innumerable years to adopt a change in man's early diet which predominantly consisted of vegetables and proteins. Refined carbohydrates and excess of fats have been thought to be the main culprit in the causation of diseases of civilization like obesity, diabetes, gall stones and heart attacks.

In people suffering from dyspepsia, diarrhoea and flatulence, fat has been incriminated as the offending agent. Fat intolerance may lead to flatulent dyspepsia or symptoms and signs referable to biliary tract. So there are strong advocates of absolutely fat free diets in people suffering from such disorders.

Studies carried out at some centres have shown that people with non-functioning gall bladder but no gall stones and symptomatic of dyspepsia, heart burn, indigestion have done very well when fats were taken off completely from their diets. This practice is worth emulating by all such sufferers.

People who suffer from gall stone disease or gall bladder dyspepsia should be advised to curtail fats in their diet drastically. The rough guidelines may be laid as follows:

(i) Of meat and its products, one should mainly be taking lean meats, fish or poultry. Meats which contain unremovable fats such as bacon, sausages, frankfurters, duck meat should be avoided. Fish and chicken when taken should either be boiled or steamed. Fried meat preparations containing rich gravy are taboos.

(ii) Milk should be taken in plenty but containing less fat. Skimmed milk is preferable. Most of the varieties of cheese, creams and butter, etc. are rich sources of saturated fats and should be avoided.

(iii) Instead of ordinary bread, brown bread is preferable. Pastries, cakes and cookies be avoided.

(iv) Fresh leafy green vegetables be taken in plenty. Potatoes, sweat potato, peas, aravi, yam be avoided. Vegetables be selected from the following—cabbage, maithi, sarson, spinach, carrots, tomatoes, bitter ground (Karela), brinjal, lady fingers, mushrooms, tinda, vegetable marrow (ghia), cucumber, etc.

Of the fruits bananas, dates, grapes, mangoes, cherries, lichis, chiku and tinned fruits of all types be avoided. grape fruit, jamun, malta, oranges, mosambi, watermelon, papaya, etc. can be liberally taken. Fruit juices (orange, mosambi, jack fruit) and lime juice cordial be taken ad lib.

(v) Dried fruits, nuts and raisins, etc. are taboos for people suffering from gall bladder dyspepsia. Similarly, cakes, chocolates, pastries, sweets of all sorts, cream soups, butter or cream biscuits be avoided.

As a basic rule, all fried foods (pakoras, samosa, potato chips, etc.) be restricted.

When taking eggs only white be taken. Broiler chicken is preferable. Substantial quantities of fresh, green leafy vegetables and salads with bread be taken. Coffee intake should be limited and preferably be taken with no cream or sugar.

The need of restricting alcoholic beverages as well as sweetened drinks cannot be overemphasised.

Thus one would appreciate that all such foods (cooked meats rich in fats, fried foods, cream, gravies, etc.) which precipitate or aggravate the condition be avoided.

Large meals and those containing indigestible articles of food (raw vegetables, unripe fruit, nuts, dried fruits, alcohol, strong tea and coffee, pickles, spices and condiments, rich and heavy puddings, highly seasoned meats, etc.) be avoided since they are likely to cause dyspepsia.

All persons who are obese must reduce their weight. At the same time the person must ensure that he/she follows basic principles of eating. Meals should be small and spread over the whole day. Food should be taken slowly but well chewed. Do not hurry with your food. Take rest for sometime after taking your meals.

Ample quantities of fluids should be taken but not in excess. Drink sparingly with meals so that it does not dilute the gastric juices and proper digestion takes place. Plenty of clear sparkling water taken between meals will add sparkle to your life.

It would be a sane practice to avoid smoking or drink alcohol on empty stomach.

In fact the patient is really the right person to decide which food to take. It is by the method of trial and error that he/she can judge as to which food suits him or which disagrees.

THE PROBLEM OF 'GAS' FORMATION

10

It is said that the three common problems which always are obsessing the mind of our people are the problem of constipation, sexual neurosis and 'GAS' formation. Many people visit doctors' clinics frequently with fantastic complaints of gas formation and its travelling to the head, heart and being responsible for a number of imagined ills.

There is nothing like gas going to the brain but it means the condition of excessive gas formation in the stomach or intestines due to number of factors.

Normally the gastrointestinal tract contains relatively small quantities of gas at any one time and mostly it does not go beyond 100-150 cc in the normal fasting state. The volume of gas increases considerably when the patient has been swallowing excess of gas.

Excessive gas formation results either due to sucking or swallowing of air during consumption of foods, but in fact it is the nervous or hysterical personality who swallows lot of air and then lets it out as well. Many people, by their bad and improper habits of eating and drinking, swallow lot of air and make a number of weird noises.

A number of folklores have always ascribed gas swallowing followed by loud belching as a sure sign of tribute to good food and cooking. But aesthetically speaking, swallowing and letting out of air is not a very desirable thing.

The diet of Indian people basically is vegetarian and most of the time the foods which are fermented in the intestines by their inadequate utilisation result in excessive gas formation.

The amount of gas in the abdomen which comes mainly from the process of swallowing air is quite large, yet gases produced by the bacterial action also form a major proportion of gas in the abdomen.

There may be abnormal bacterial flora in the intestines and the gas formation and its amount will vary with the type of bacteria and the variety of substances on which they grow. These are further influenced by the contents of food stuff eaten, bacterial flora, stasis in the intestines, acidity in the stomach and the time taken by the food to travel in the intestines.

It is said that more than 50 to 70 per cent of the gas in the abdomen comes from air that has been swallowed. Excess air is swallowed as a result of bad habits of eating, excessive belching and in the act of swallowing of more saliva and then air. A form of subconscious reaction due to tension, anxiety or grief may be there which leads to the habit of swallowing more air.

Similarly, people who suffer from ulcers, the constant dyspepsia of which they are victims, may induce belching as a form of habit.

In addition, excessive smoking, poor hygiene of the mouth and excessive use of carbonated drinks and beer are all contributory factors towards the malady. Faulty habits of eating contribute in no way in lesser manner towards aggravating the problem. People who do not eat their food properly and have the habit of gulping food rapidly or bolting it down with lot of water or fluids in between the meals also suffer from excessive gas formation. Normally a little amount of air is swallowed along with food or drink but when eating rapidly, increased amount of air is swallowed. Similarly, mouth breathers, fast eaters also swallow lot of air and in the latter category no time is given to the stomach to adjust itself to the food.

Some people take carbonated drinks to get relief from gas but in fact they unknowingly increase the amount of gas inside their tummy. At the same time some people knowingly swallow air to induce belching because on some previous occasion the person had experienced some relief from the distressing gas with eructations. Thus relief obtained once may lead to the habit of regular belching and an undesirable habit of belching and letting out of gas may be formed. But actually these people are swallowing more of air.

There may be abnormal bacterial flora in the intestines and the gas formation and its amount will vary with the type of bacterial flora and the variety of substances on which they grow. These are further influenced by the contents of food stuff eaten, stasis in the intestines, acidity in the stomach and the time taken by the food to travel in the intestines.

It is not easy to change the intestinal tract flora and food especially consisting of large quantities of inadequately cooked or cellulose fibres may give rise to the production of excess gas serving as a good medium for the growth of bacteria. In this category fall diets containing excess of starch, and food traditionally labelled as gas formers include pulses, legumes, beans, cabbage, onions, cauliflower, radishes, cucumber, potatoes beetroot and celery. Flatus is also markedly increased by apple and grape juices, raisins and bananas. Spicy fried food and condiments further aggravate gas formation. Some people suffer from a form of carbohydrate dyspepsia where excessive formation, belching, borborygmi (noises in the abdomen) result due to intolerance to starches.

Taking of diet containing excess of leafy and fibrous vegetables like salads, may also result in excessive gas formation and passage. There are number of examples in the animal kingdom which will illustrate this point better. Take the example of herbivorous animals, e.g., horses etc. and consider the food being consumed by it. No wonder such animals are always letting out lot of gas.

In the normal course the gas produced in the abdomen is odorless but when it is passed out it contains lot of undesirable odor which makes passing of gas very much aesthetically undesirable.

The main constituents of the gas are nitrogen, carbon dioxide (produced by the fermentative reactions between organic acids and bicarbonates), hydrogen (derived mainly from bacterial metabolic processes), methane, oxygen and trace gases.

Nitrogen, carbon dioxide, hydrogen, methane and oxygen are non-odorous gases and it is the trace gases which account for the unpleasant odour of the flatus. This comes from ammonia, hydrogen sulphide, indole, mercaptane, volatile amines and short chain fatty acids.

In addition to the factor of swallowing of excess of air, faulty eating habits, one should not forget the role of parasites in the intestines to which Indian people suffer very frequently not only because of lack of sanitation facilities but also due to improper hygienic habits. The incidence of parasitic infestations and amoebiasis is probably the highest in our population and this contributes to a large extent in the production of excessive gas formation as well as sense of distension in the abdomen. Excessive or low acidity may be another important cause which may be due to either inflammation of lower end of food pipe or stomach or regurgitation of food. When acidity is present in excess, factors responsible may be: more use of alcoholic drinks, smoking, aspirin, pickles, chutnis, spices, etc. Similarly, excessive fermentation and putrefaction of food in the intestines may be as a result of abnormal bacterial flora, deficiency of enzymes and diseases of the intestines including milk intolerance. So apparently gas formation is not necessarily due to a single factor but a number of factors.

Excessive gas formation and letting it out is not an aesthetically desirable proposition and is always a constant source of stress on the mind of layman. Most of these people are seen complaining of excessive and frequent belching, growling or rumbling noises in the abdomen, a sense of bloating or distension.

Naturally the question arises as to how to manage this problem? In the management of such people there are broad principles. First of all one must exclude any disease process in the abdomen which could be accounting for excessive gas formation. These include chronic disease of pancreas, ulcers in the stomach, disease of the intestines associated with foul smelling stools, flatulent diarrhoea associated with intolerance to milk and parasitic infestations.

At the same time one should keep note of the person's method of eating whether food eaten hurriedly or not chewed properly. Some people may be addicted to gum chewing, excessive smoking or making frequent use of soda tablets or carbonated beverages.

In the second category are people who have got a predominant psychogenic background coupled with anxiety and hysterical predisposition. These are the people who have got what is called a 'gaseous personality'. If one listens patiently to such people one would appreciate that they have got the most bizarre sort of complaints. They are emotionally labile, have got a fixation complex about the excessive gas and probably will ascribe all their complaints of ill health to the gas formation. Such people require a thorough psychiatric assessment and invariably the doctors are able to pinpoint some psychological or hysterical background to the problem. Even for a laymen it is not difficult to recognise such people. They are belching very loudly, making odd noises and bringing out lot of air through the mouth. One has often observed even whistling sounds emanating from such people. People who suffer from such ailment should be sympathised and dealt with in condescending manner rather than that fun is made of them. With the help of a psychiatrist and physician coupled with proper explanation and understanding of the problem a lot of success can be achieved in alleviating the sufferings of such people.

In the third category are people who do not present with bizarre symptoms but always complain of excessive gas formation.

In such group of people the causes may be many. One cannot lay down mathematical rules to follow in such people but broad guidelines may be given. The person may not be chewing the food properly and may be rather wolfing down the food hurriedly. Some people have got the faulty habit of swallowing air while eating or drinking so first advice should be to cultivate saner eating habits.

The person must take small morsels of food, chew them properly and should not try to hurry down the food. Food should be taken in small portions and more frequently rather than gulping down big helpings of food at one sitting. Water or fluids should not be taken with meals but only after the food, since taking of water during meals may distend the stomach and interfere with the digestion of food by its diluting effect on the gastric juices. Food must be taken at regular hours and not in an irregular manner.

Avoid hurry at the dinner table and take food at a leisurely pace. Evening meals should not be taken immediately after coming from work but preferably take them after resting for atleast half an hour or so. Take your meals in a quiet peaceful atmosphere. Let the dining table be not the venue for discussions of all the unpleasant events of the day.

People who are accustomed to either gum chewing, sucking on ciagars or excessive smoking must cut on them.

Avoid carbonated drinks, beer, milk shakes, etc. since they produce more gas.

Diet must be clean, light and properly planned. Foods which are known to produce excessive gas like starches, potatoes, beans, cabbage, cauliflower, cucumber, radishes, turnips, root vegetables, lentils like urad dal, etc. be cut down. It does not in any way mean that we should not consume wheat, rice or potatoes, etc. One would prefer that whole wheat flour rather than white flour, and unpolished rice instead of polished rice be substituted in the diet.

People who suffer from dyspepsia due to carbohydrates have to cut on their starch diet and take comparatively less of starch. In their diet potatoes, beetroots, green peas, rajma, puddings, pastries and sweets should be reduced.

Too much of spicy and fried rich food, thick gravies and foods cooked with excess fat are always a source of dyspepsia and gas formation, so cut on them. Intake of apple juice, grape juice and excess of raw fruit vegetables be cut.

Over-eating especially at parties must be checked. Omission of soup or fruit juice with the night meal will help. Plan a well proportioned and balanced diet containing all nutrients in proper proportions. Even taking of excessive delicacies of non-vegetarian diet may produce putrefaction and undesirable gases. So take meat preparations preferably steamed or cooked with less spices and fats.

Salads are good and their use is recommended for the maintenance of normal bowel action. But when people start consuming them in excess, that is where the trouble occurs.

Food items which are rich in refined sugars like pastries, chocolates, sweat meats produce fermentation, so if you suffer from gas problem, cut on them.

Have a diet containing fresh vegetables, fruits but less of starch, condiments and soft foods.

When deficiency of enzymes in intestines is suspected (Doctor is the best judge in this matter) taking of enzyme preparations after each principal meal helps.

If increased acidity is present then cut on your smoke, alcohol and spices. Use of antacids also helps.

Avoid constipation but at the same time avoid the use of laxatives. Ensure regularity of bowels.

Preferably take your food in loose clothes. Avoid tight-fitting clothes at dinner time. Have a leisurely stroll after your evening meal. Do not lie down in bed or slump in an easy chair immediately after taking food, since doing so will aggravate the feeling of distension in abdomen.

Lastly when talking about the problem of gas, let us not ignore the fact that there may be some organic diseases like parasites in the intestines, ulcer in the stomach or even an obstruction in the stomach which might be responsible for the production of excessive gas. People who suffer from excessive gas may also be constipated. This might be due to number of factors like lack of exercise, use of only refined foodstuffs or soft foods and lack of training in toilet habits. Where constipation is the responsible factor, it must be corrected and remedied. Use of purgatives in constipation is not a very desirable thing. Attempts should be made to educate the patient on diet, exercise and if necessary some mild laxative like isogel (isabgol) at bed time is advised.

Most of the people in our country suffer from amoebic infection which is a very important cause of indigestion and gas formation. This must be treated with proper medication. At the same time when worms in the intestines are suspected the person has to be 'de-wormed'.

Patient with problem of excessive gas formation must be investigated for parasitic infestations, pancreatic disease and ulcer. One should look for acidity since both hyperacidity and low acidity may be responsible. Stools should be examined for parasites and undigested food particles. Culture of intestinal contents is sometimes required to find the type of bacteria present. Some people may require Barium Meal Study of stomach and duodenum to exclude presence of ulcer.

In fact besides various factors about eating habits and life style etc., one must exclude any organic disease, if present.

To conclude, excessive formation of gas is a problem which troubles the layman a lot and it has got both psychogenic, dietic as well as organic factors as being responsible. The correct management means understanding the psyche of the patient, correction of faulty eating habits and treatment of the organic diseases, if any. Given the correct approach it should not be difficult problem to manage.

TUMMY UPSET

11

Tummy upset is a common problem from which most of the people suffer at sometime or the other. A lot of people are chronic sufferer from this malady and many often become nervous wrecks because of their long drawn-out tummy problems. It is not difficult to come across lot of such people in one's day to day practice.

For example, take the case of Mr. A. He is all the time complaining of vague abdominal discomfort, sense of distension or gas formation, excessive passage of wind and often peculiar sounds in the abdomen. Otherwise he looks to be in the prime of health yet he remains morose and often depressed since he feels that the charms of life are being denied to him because of his abdominal upsets which make him irritable, quarrelsome and short-tempered. Let us look at the problems of Mr. A. He is a travelling salesman and though earns substantially well, yet his food habits are rather one which leave much to be desired. He often indulges in round of parties, is always in a hurry to move. So gulps his food and unfortunately is very fond of rich fried foods. Moreover, his meal hours are irregular and because of the nature of his job he has to take food from hotels and dhabas almost half the month.

The other case is that of Mrs. B, a sedate housewife, whose family life is rather unhappy and she is always under great tension. Moreover, she is very fond of achars, chutneys and spices. The result is that though she remains high-strung all the time, yet she feels always out of sorts because of her stomach. She often complains of discomfort during or soon after meals; mostly it is like a heartburn and there is abdominal fullness. She has often sought treatment from the local 'Churans' or indigenous drugs but the results have been rather unsatisfactory. In fact she is all the time worried over her indigestion.

The above are just two examples of the type of people who come complaining of tummy upsets.

Tummy upset generally means indigestion and it may be seen in many forms. It is rather a vague, ill-defined term and its presentations can be most varied and bizarre. A person may have a sense of heaviness or distension in abdomen, belching, discomfort either during, immediately or at varying periods after meals. Some may suffer from a sense of being unwell, loss of appetite or fear of getting discomfort after eating which may keep them away from food.

A typical person who suffers from indigestion is not especially fat or thin, young or old, harassed or clam but has a typical personality. He has some discomfort, during or soon after meals. It may be in the form of heartburn, belching, abdominal fullness and discomfort. A person is aware of these spells of indigestion and generally is self treating with much advertised remedies.

It is the persistence of these symptoms which brings him to the doctor. People who suffer from tummy upsets often become irritable or depressed and have a quarrelsome personality and become jittery. A number of factors are operative in the causation of indigestion and these range from faulty eating habits, unhygienic food, improper toilet habits, lack of physical exercise and mental tension to diseases of stomach (gastritis, ulcer), intestines (worm infestation, amoebiasis), liver and gall bladder dysfunction and lastly cancer of the gastrointestinal tract.

Of the faulty eating habits being an important cause of tummy upset, there are no two views about it. Overeating at home or more commonly at parties, feasts, marriages and partaking of rich, greasy food at such occasions is a common way of life with most people. Again, it is not only the excessive consumption of food but also the type of food partaken which has a bearing on the problem. Most of the times the food is of rich quality, fried and excessively spiced, containing lot of fats and other ingredients which go a long way in making the person uncomfortable as the rich oily food is difficult to digest.

Another common problem with our people is the habit of consuming food from wayside hotels and dhabas. One does not want to outright condemn such establishments but the one where the standards of hygiene and cleanliness leave much to be desired. The food may be stale, cooked in unhygienic surroundings and the servant/cook may not be maintaining proper standards of personal hygiene.

Similarly, raw cut foods and fruits sold on wayside *rehris* are a constant source of infection leading to abdominal upset. At the same time we must keep in mind the unhygienic habits of cook/servant at home. Stale, left-over, under-cooked and food over-rich in fats has to be avoided. It is not only the food but due attention has to be paid to the cleanliness of kitchen and clean, pure water supply. Many ills of people in our country are due to impure water supply. Worm infestation, loose motions due to use of infected food or unclean water supply are common bug bears of tummy upset. A word about amoebiasis which is so common in our country that more than 90 per cent of the population suffer from it and a very constant source of tummy upset and ill health. In our country almost every other person has either suffered or is suffering from amoebiasis and it may run in families. The organism gains entrance into the body via the oral route either through infected water or food. When passed in stools it has the properties of being resistant to the surroundings and can live for 10 days outside. Boiling of water containing the parasite kills it. Many persons who suffer from the disease pass the cysts of the parasite in their stools and become a source of chronic infection.

Toilet habits of most of our people leave much to be desired. Most of the poorer sections of society do not have proper latrines in their homes and even those who have, do not observe proper hygiene. It is a common site to see people defecating on the roadside, in the fields and near water reservoirs like ponds, canals, rivers, etc. This results in infection of water which when used for irrigation of fields leads to the infection of vegetables which when eaten raw results in infection. Similarly, practice of using human waste as manure in fields further perpetuates the spread of amoebiasis. Flies and cockroaches are other important source of conveying infection from infected stools to the food and water. But the most important place in this whole drama goes to personal hygiene not only of self but also of cook in the house who handles the food. When amoeba attacks the person, a common complaint is tummy upset, flatulence, heartburn chronic ill health and irregular bowel habits.

Children and even adults who suffer from worms in their intestines are often complaining of tummy upset. Some may even see worms in their stools on naked eye.

Tummy upset causes include a wide spectrum. People who do not devote adequate time for their food and are always in a hurry to gulp down the food and come to the dining table loaded with worries either of home or office often suffer from indigestion. Such people who are either angry, worried or depressed in them not only the secretions of their stomach essential for proper digestion are depressed but their food is not properly assimilated.

If food can be an important factor responsible for indigestion then how it is eaten and way it is eaten are equally important factors. Eating of food properly is also an act which has to be cultivated. Very few people observe regular meal hours. People living in big cities who have to commute to far off places from their residences to place of work or busy professionals whose very nature of work demands a great strain on their time, the regularity of meal times is rather difficult to observe. Irregularity of timings of meals shall not only pull the normal body responses to food but shall also affect the gastric secretions. The sum total of this is indigestion.

Then it is equally important to chew the food properly and not to take big morsels and lot of fluids in between the meals as these shall dilute gastric secretion. Fluids should preferably be taken after meals. Improperly chewed food which has not been allowed to mix with saliva in the mouth shall not be properly digested. People who consume large amount of spices, condiments, pickles, chutneys, etc. and make excessive use of strong tea, coffee, alcohol or smoke are liable to suffer from tummy upset or indigestion.

If the cleanliness of food is important then the mental state of the individual is equally important. Lack of sleep due to long hours of work or under periods of stress shall result in the disturbances of normal physiological processes where appetite for food is lost, bowels are not opened and the person suffers from indigestion. Spices, condiments, pickles and chutneys constitute an important ingredient of diet of our people. Excessive use of these causes irritation of the gastric mucosa resulting in discomfort and indigestion. Tea and coffee are enjoyable beverages but it is their improper preparation, i.e., taking too strong or consumption in excess and on empty stomach is an important offender in irritating the stomch mucosa. The person complains of burning sensation in the pit of stomach, lack of appetite and is a constant sufferer from indigestion.

Alcoholic drinks and excessive smoking coupled with the habit of tobacco chewing are also important causes of indigestion. People who take either undiluted alcohol (neat peg), adulterated spurious variety and in excess and often on empty stomach at the same time ignoring need for proper nutrition become sufferer from indigestion almost for their lifetime. To start with, this is due to irritation of gastric mucosa as a result of direct injury from alcohol but later on the alcohol affects the liver with the result that not only the stomach cease to function properly but also the liver. Smokers also suffer from abdominal discomfort and often complain of either pain in abdomen or loss of appetite. This is as a result of the effect of nicotine and smoke on gastric secretions.

Leading an active physical life in contrast to a life of laziness and slothfulness or a sedentary existence also contribute towards tilting or untilting the balance of digestion.

An active individual is always able to move his bowels regularly. People who have a feeling of dissatisfaction with their bowel movement or have the habit of voiding stools several times a day and have an urge to go again always have a feeling of discomfort in the abdomen. Lack of bowel movements or in other words constipation takes away greater part of an individual's time. Though a number of factors ranging from hygiene of the toilet to the type of foods and vegetables being consumed may be responsible for sluggish bowels, yet a layman most of the time is not satisfied till he has moved his bowels at least once in a day and in adequate quantities. Poor bowel movements always produce funny ideas in people's mind. They feel listless, unwell, loose their appetite and complain of indigestion.

In short, the causes of indigestion for which no structural cause can be demonstrated depend to a large extent on either physical or mental stress which affects the alimentary system. People who are of either sensitive nature or who keep their emotions bottled up are much more liable to become victims to it. In this regard physical rest has also been given lot of importance. People who are always on the go and travelling from place to place too frequently are very often the victims of indigestion. That is why it is desirable to take some rest after a principal meal. Last but not least, let us not ignore a very important facet of the habit of people who suffer from indigestion. Some people are habituated to the use of painkillers like Aspirin and Laxatives due to high powered advertisements all over the world both via radio and news media. These people are often an easy prey to indigestion. Of all these functional causes the silver-lining is that little effort on the part of the individuals can go a long way in correcting the indigestion.

But difficulty arises when indigestion is due to some organic cause in the alimentary tract and number of diseases starting from food pipe (oesophagus) to large gut (colon) to liver and gall bladder can cause indigestion. When talking about organic causes of indigestion for the layman one must at the outset clarify that it is rather a complicated subject, since it encompasses a number of diseases of diverse aetiology which are best left in the hands of the treating physician for diagnosis and management.

Oesophagitis (inflammation of food pipe) is a common condition associated with either intake of hot, spicy food and heavy meals, excessive intake of alcoholic beverages. It commonly occurs in people who immediately retire to bed after a bout of heavy food. Sometimes, there is obstruction or dysfunction of the lower end of oesophageal sphincter and rarely a cancer of oestophagus. There is loss of appetite and difficulty in swallowing food.

Hiatus hernia is another condition in which a portion of stomach or oesophagus protrudes through the opening at the lower end of oesophagus in diaphragm and is in the form of a sliding or gliding hernia. Hiatus hernia may be present for long but symptoms become apparent only later on in life. Most of such people feel uncomfortable when lying in bed after meals and often complain of a sense of heaviness either behind the breast bone (sternum) or of dyspepsia. The symptoms in such people are worsened after consumption of heavy, rich food wearing of tight clothes or garters especially if the sufferer is fat or when such people bend forward after taking meals. Another common complaint is a feeling of regurgitation of food and food eaten earlier on gives an unpleasant taste. This may be only an indication of indigestion but when persists means that there is some obstruction lower down.

Feeling of water brash, i.e., the filling of mouth with tasteless fluid like saliva may occur repeatedly in nervous individuals but may occur sometimes in people with either gastritis or ulcer in the stomach.

Stomach is one organ which probably plays a very important role as the villain of the story of indigestion. Stomach has the capacity to adapt to its maximum to the variations in the food habit of the individual ranging from all types of exotic, sweet, hot, rich, spicy foods to variegated nature of beverages including alcoholic drinks. But there are people who are allergic to certain foods which include milk, fish, eggs, etc. whose consumption in very minor quantity sets up a chain reaction of discomfort, belly ache and indigestion.

Then again contaminated stale food or improperly cooked food are a great source of indigestion. Inflammation of stomach (gastritis) may be either acute or of long duration (chronic). Chronic gastritis is generally due to consumption of spicy foods, hot tea or coffee, smoking and alcohol for over long periods. There is generally pain, nausea, loss of appetite.

Cancer of the stomach is rather a dangerous condition and is often missed to start with, since it starts rather vaguely; patient often complains of slight discomfort in the upper part of abdomen, indigestion and loss of appetite. The patient generally an elderly individual starts complaining of weakness and gradually weight loss sets in, since the appetite is now being gradually lost. What started with mild discomfort and got relieved by taking some "Churan" or digestant tablet now fails to be relieved by such home remedies and by the time the possibility of such a disease is considered or the patient goes to the doctor, probably it is too late. It only means that if any person beyond the age of 45 years starts either loosing weight or complains of dyspepsia it is time to look up.

Ulcer in the stomach or duodenum has got a very specific pattern and the pain has got specific relationship with food. There is a burning sensation in the epigastric region and most of the times the individual has been getting relief by taking soda mint tablets or some soda bicarb drink. Pain at times is severe. In case of gastric ulcer the pain is increased by taking of food and is relieved after the food has passed down, while pain in duodenal ulcer comes two to three hours after taking food. In fact food relieves pain. But pain in both cases is relieved by taking either milk or alkalis. The pain may be dull, boring or penetrating type. It is the chronicity of pain and failure of relief by the use of much advertised mint tablets which brings the person to the doctor.

Intestinal diseases both of small as well as large are important causes of indigestion. Worm infestations, diarrhoeas due to use of contaminated food or unclean water supply or amoebic infection are very common bug bears of ill health and indigestion. Amoebic dysentery either acute or chronic is very prevalent in our country and probably more than ninety per cent of our population suffers from it in some form or the other. Chronic amoebic infection is a very common cause of indigestion, flatulence, belching and chronic ill health.

Traveller's diarrhoea, tropical sprue, non-tropical sprue, tuberculosis of the intestines and cancer are other important causes to be considered. There is one more intestinal condition in contrast to constipation where a person has always a desire to go again and a sense of dissatisfaction about the emptying of bowels. This is known as irritable bowel. Constipation is one condition which is probably considered by a layman to be the root cause of all indigestion he/she may be suffering from. Most of such people suffer from a constant ill health, bad tempers, headache, flatulence and dyspepsia.

But indigestion does not mean only diseases or ailments confined either to stomach, duodenum, small or large intestines. Gall bladder dyspepsia especially of chronic form is very common in fat females and is important cause of indigestion, flatulence and distaste for heavy, rich foods. Liver is one organ which plays a major part in maintaining digestion. People suffering from chronic liver diseases are victims of indigestion almost for the lifetime. Any acute inflammation of liver (Hepatitis) gives rise to loss of appetite and indigestion to start with. Chronic alcoholic suffers from indigestion not only because of inflammation of stomach (Gastritis) but also due to inflammation and damage of liver.

Pancreas (or sweet bread) is another important organ which has a role to play in maintaining proper digestion because of its secretions. So diseases of pancreas ranging from pancreatitis to cancer are important causes responsible for indigestion. List of conditions causing indigestion is unending. Inflammation of peritoneum, formation of adhesions, renal failure, severe anaemia, diseases of the ductless glands, pulmonary tuberculosis, chronic use of any drug, for that matter, common home remedies like aspirin, tonics, etc. all give rise to indigestion and it is for the treating doctor to make a diagnosis. For the layman it is important to keep in mind that any indigestion which lasts for a few days and is a source of nuisance, requires looking into.

How to Look for Indigestion?

If you suffer from indigestion then it is very important for you to understand certain guidelines which should help you in salvaging the problem. As one physician wrote , "indigestion is a meaningless term for what may be meaningful symptoms." Similarly, one has to appreciate that the use of term is rather being made indiscriminately for host of minor and even sometimes serious complaints. The first question to ask oneself is to what bothers you the most? It is just a sensation of burning heat or warmth in the upper abdomen or that air is being sucked in the stomach while drinking or eating food, resulting in a sense of bloating and gaseousness. These are the very people who may be very much high strung and belch loudly. It is not difficult to appreciate as to why these people suffer from indigestion, gaseousness, passage of flatus and too frequent noisy belching. The real villain in all this is probably the person concerned himself, since he has bad eating habits and gulps down his food too rapidly and is rather fond of either taking too much of carbonated drinks or excessive amounts of fluids with the food. Then again certain foods like beans, milk, pastries, chocolates, cakes and rich, fried foods produce excessive gaseous distension due to improper digestion because of either putrefaction or lack of proper fermentation.

Some people are swallowing too much air, belching loudly and then when they bloat up, they blame some imaginary illness. So ask yourself—Do you suffer from gaseous indigestion? If so is it the way you eat your food or take your drinks a responsible factor? Can you correct it. The second important question is—what foods do not suit you? Do you suffer from intolerance to certain foods like milk, fish, eggs, etc. Make up an inventory of foods eaten during the last 24-48 hours and many a time you shall be able to pinpoint the food item which is the main culprit for your indigestion. Think of the places like wayside restaurants, hotels or dhabas or a feast you might have attended during the last 24-48 hours and you shall know the cause of indigestion. Next in line of self-questioning is as to how long the indigestion has been present? A recently developed indigestion points towards a recent cause but when the indigestion has persisted for long periods then it is time to go to your doctor. Let us not forget that indigestion results not only from abdominal diseases but also from diseases in other systems like heart, kidney, lungs and even for that reason in the nervous system. In females mensturation, pregnancy, all are very specifically related to digestive disturbances like nausea, vomiting, heartburn and indigestion.

But if indigestion means loss of appetite and progressive loss of weight then it is time to sit up and think of more serious ailments and for that reason even cancer in the gastrointestinal tract.

In elderly people indigestion may be due to lack of acid in the gastric juice but when pallor and anaemia supervenes, it means that there is some source of bleed from the gastrointestinal tract. Lastly, ask yourself whether you remain tense, anxious or depressed. Psyche has great influence over the digestion of the individual. It is possible that you are harbouring either an overt allergy or distaste to certain foods and subconsciously you suffer from indigestion. Emotional stress and strain have a definite bearing on the appetite and digestive functions.

One cannot ignore the fact that drug abuse, alcohol addiction and smoking all have got an indirect bearing to the frustrations and tensions of everyday life and no wonder these abuses directly and indirectly contribute to the production of dyspepsia and indigestion.

Investigations of Indigestion

Since indigestion is so common a thing, every person suffering from indigestion does not require detailed investigations. Most of the time people suffering from dyspepsia require tackling of the basic disease itself and once it is done so, satisfactory results can be achieved.

In a majority of people simple advice about hygiene of food and water helps. A stools examination is a must in every case, since a large number of population in our country suffers from parasitic infestations.

If the preliminary investigations do not help then one has to take recourse to further detailed tests like gastric acidity test, X-ray studies of stomach, duodenum, small intestines and gall bladder and endoscopic examination of the gastrointestinal tract by the use of flexible fibreoptic instruments. Occasionally, biopsies are taken from the stomach, duodenum and liver for further confirmation of the diagnosis. But let us not forget that indigestion can be due to a wide range of diseases of the gastrointestinal tract both functional and organic as well as of other systems in the body and the doctor is the best judge to advise the future line of diagnosis and management.

The problem of excessive gas formation can be avoided by taking clean wholesome food and not partaking of rich fried foods, confectionery like sweets and chocolates, etc. But all the above measures are only general principles and for any organic disease responsible for tummy upset, treating physician is the best guide. For diseases and dysfunctions of the tummy upset, appropriate measures must be taken.

How to Manage Tummy Upset

We have briefly described common cause of tummy upset. Though an occasional tummy upset can be managed by a layman yet in long drawn-out cases it is better left in the hands of a competent physician who shall properly investigate and reach appropriate diagnosis with subsequent management. Let us look at some of the general principles which may help a lay person suffering from tummy upset.

Since most of the time tummy upset is the result of over-eating and almost with the principle of "No Control" over the palate, so best is to eat and restrict your food to a little less than your appetite. In other words "Do not overfeed". Let lavish parties and dinners be not a part of your daily living. Keep a control over yourself. It is not that one is advising a person to be a social outcast and avoid social functions and parties. One can always be a successful social go-getter if you restrict your food intake to only as per your daily requirement. Avoid rich, spicy foods which are laden with too much 'grease' or fat. Excess of sweets be avoided, since rich confectionery can produce too much gas. Avoid excessive use of pickled and spicy foods. Cultivate the habit of taking simple clean foods which are nourishing and easy to digest. Excess of beverages like alcohol, beer, tea, coffee and colas be avoided. Very hot drink shall produce a form of inflammation of the stomach, so control the intake of very hot foods or scalding drinks.

There can be no two views about taking care of not partaking foods which are prepared in unhygienic conditions. So look around when taking eatables from wayside joints. Most of the time the water supply is infected and many infections are conveyed through it. So see to it that water used for drinking purposes is pure and clean. Best way to ensure clean water supply is to boil the water for 10-15 minutes, cool it and then use for drinking purposes.

The most important factor is to cultivate clean personal habits. Proper learning of toilet hygiene must be ensured. Have regular bowel habits. This can be achieved by leading an active life, avoidance of soft refined food and adequate use of fresh fruits, vegetables and salads. All vegetables and fruits must be washed thoroughly before cooking and eating raw.

If you are one of those busy persons who is always having a round of parties then it calls for a break in the schedule. A week end of simple food fare at home shall give a much needed rest to your digestive system.

Do not take drugs unnecessarily. Every person who suffers from indigestion does not necessarily have high acidity. In fact low acidity is an equally important cause of dyspepsia. In persons with high acidity antacids help, while in those with low acidity antacids shall rather harm than do good.

If a person is fond of his "Chhota peg" and cannot leave it off, he should not only cut the intake of alcohol but there should be at least interval for period of 24 hours between two sessions of drinks. Interval free period gives rest to the liver, gives it time to recover from injury and minimise the damage.

Let not worry and hurry be watchword at meal time. Have small periods of rest after every main meal. Chew your food properly and take small morsels. Do not gulp the food. Keep worry, anxiety and mental tension at bay at meal time. If you have to catch a train, bus or plane or go on an important engagement then leave time enough for yourself to take food in peaceful atmosphere. Let phone be kept away at meal time. There cannot be anything worse then repeated interruptions at meal time.

Food should be taken in a relaxed state of mind and with pleasure, joy and a sense of satisfaction. Many people just start fretting at the dining-table at the site of some dish which is not to their liking. Emotions like anxiety, anger, depression effect the secretions of stomach. So, have control on your emotions.

In other words tummy upset which can be very distressing can be managed if adequate precautions are taken about eating habits, personal and general hygiene, ensuring clean and pure water supply as well as proper thrust on the factors responsible for tummy upset.

12 CONSTIPATION — MODERN AGE AILMENT

It is said that modern civilization has brought in its wake a situation where the affluent have developed a sweet tooth, discarded the habit of exercise, have become dependant on modern gadgets and in return have got a number of disorders of various organs. In this list one important place may be given to "constipation" which is defined as a dysfunction where the bowels are emptied at long intervals with or without difficulty.

The incidence of constipation in general population is variable. Studies all over the world have shown that a number of normal people pass one or two motions a day and this is considered as natural while more than three bowel actions per day may be considered as abnormal. The range of so-called normal values also differ. While an Indian may not be satisfied with the passage of one motion a day, his counterpart in the West may be satisfied even with moving his bowels only three times a week.

Majority of people are always obsessed with the number and frequency of their bowel action and often exhibit a sense of overconcern. Often there is a feeling of abnormality in that either the amount of stool passed is too little or there is a sense of inadequate evacuation.

The frequency of bowel action depends to a large extent on the nature and type of diet being consumed by the people. Thus in our country where the staple diet contains more roughage and is greater in quantity as well as bulk, the stools are large and bulky as compared to the Western people whose diet is more refined and soft, the stools are rather small and infrequent. The mores differ. As already alluded to, in Western society even if a person does not pass motion for two days it may be considered as normal, while with Indian people passing of one motion may be considered inadequate. So, one would appreciate that what may be considered as normal bowel action for one group of people may not be so for others. The problem of constipation is global, though it is more a disease of civilization rather than of primitive communities.

Basically, constipation is directly related to the act of defecation which is dependant on number of factors like the area of bowel distended, the rate and amount of pressure being exerted and anatomical as well as nervous integrity of the nerves supplying the anus and rectum. This mechanism, though apparently a complex one, is an efficient but flexible one and goes on rather uninterruptedly.

Nature has made everything so mechanical and automatic that the process of absorption, storing and finally expulsion of residual unabsorbed foodstuffs goes on in a regular manner. But any small dysfunction in this mechanism brings home to us the significance of healthy and normal bowel movements.

Bowel action normally is stimulated by ingestion of food and physical activity. Thus it is a common practice that on getting up in the morning when a person moves about, a form of propulsive movement of the intestine takes place with resultant evacuation. Similarly, eating effects the motility of the colon. Taking of food starts a form of gastrocolic reflex. Many people have a close relationship between eating and the desire to defecate. But the propulsive action of bowels is further facilitated by the use of bed tea or drinking of water in the morning.

But it is the sluggishness of bowel action which worries an individual and produces a sense of being unwell. In contrast to it, on the other side, all people who pass motion only two or three times a week and remain constipated but still may be comfortable and have no sense of ill health, while in the former category of people there is always a feeling of discomfort not only of the abdomen and body but also a feeling of being unwell.

The problem of constipation from the viewpoint of a layman is really enormous, since a number of symptoms of ill health are always ascribed to this malady.

Most of the complaints are either limited to infrequency of bowel action or to a feeling of inadequate evacuation or of passing a too hard stool with difficulty. Superimposed over it are features of anxiety, a feeling of being constantly suffering from ill health due to inadequate bowel action and many of such individuals have got complaints bordering on a 'neurotic personality'.

Causes of Constipation

There are innumerable reasons why a person can be a victim of constipation.

Many times the constipation may be self-induced due to food fads of the individual, intake of foods which are primarily soft and are devoid of roughage and fibre. In our country lack of fluids also contributes to a large extent in inducing constipation, since body loses large amounts of fluids from perspiration and if adequate quantities of appropriate fluids are not taken, the stools may become dry and hard with resultant constipation.

Faulty food intake holds the prime importance for being a responsible factor. This not only includes inadequate intake of food but also irregular hours of meals and taking of soft, non-bulk forming foods like pizzas, pastries, cakes, puddings, etc.

Our ancestors have always stressed the importance of roughage in food or high fibre containing foods. In fact it is the way of life with people in less developed societies. But in the more affluent West the food basically is soft, non-bulk forming. Even during the last hundred years Western people have registered an enormous increase in their consumption of refined sugars, white flour products as well as non-bulk producing foods. Use of confectionary and soft foods is an accepted way of life with the Westerns.

High refined and soft foods predispose the Western to pass stools which are smaller and less frequent. There is a disturbance of the regulatory mechanisms of the gut and the result is not only constipation but also other innumerable health hazards.

There is no doubt that the removal of unabsorbable fibre in the modern foodstuffs has got profound effect on the stool bulk and content. Use of non-bulk forming foods delays the transit time of the contents in colon with resultant constipation. The effects of high roughage diet is well demonstrated amongst communities in Africa where two or three bowel actions take place daily.

Dietary fibre is an unimportant source of energy but is now being recognized to play a significant part in the diet of humans and an essential substance of maintaining the health of the gut. It consists of substances of plant material resistant to digestion, predominantly comprising of cellulose, hemicellulose and a non-carbohydrate substance.

Adding fibre containing foods to the diet increases faecal bulk and improves bowel habits. At the same time, the time taken for food residual to pass through the gut is shortened by dietary fibre. This is because high fibre containing foods have good water binding capacity or bulking properties and by carrying food wastes in fast transit, it increases the process of evacuation of the gut.

Apparently the role of diet *vis-à-vis* constipation cannot be minimized and one has to appreciate that in majority of people the main factor responsible is faulty dietary habits.

Next to food being a prime factor, lack of physical activity, exercise, leading a sedentary life and a life dependent on push button gadgets—all predispose to the development of constipation. People who lead an active outdoor life and take part in active sports rarely complain of bowel dysfunction.

It is equally important to cultivate the habit of going regularly in the morning to the bathroom from the very childhood. Ignoring the call to pass stool if cultivated regularly is likely to be an important cause of factors contributing towards constipation.

Similarly, inadequate time early in the morning when the call occurs, hurrying up, poor toilet facilities, too much travel all will contribute towards disturbing the normal cycle of bowel movements. Apparently, regular function coupled with regular habits will go a long way in preventing the development of bowel neurosis.

It has also been pointed out that the position adopted while defecating may have an important bearing to the problem and the ideal position is the squatting position. Since western type of toilet may be too high and feet may dangle with the result that the muscles which play part in aiding the act of defecation have little opportunity to fulfil their functions, so it is advised that people who remain constipated they should avoid the bed pan and whenever possible a commode be employed or the squatting position on Indian type of toilet be preferred.

Next important factor is emotions. It has been said that colon is the image of our emotions. Nothing can be more true than this. Emotions have lot of role to play in the control of normal bowel movements. In states of depression the gut activity is inhibited and constipation results. Since not only there is poor intake of food but also a generalized sluggishness. At the same time spasm of the gut takes place under mental tension.

In the same category let us not forget people who are addicted to purgatives. These are the people who are obsessed with their bowel movements and have always a feeling of inadequate emptying. Such person often are in the habit of taking strong purgatives regularly with resultant loss of fluids and electrolytes. A form of dehydration of the gut results and there is rebound constipation which looks very much contradictory to the person, since he is already on purgatives. While referring to various factors about diet, emotions and exercise, let us not ignore a very important aspect of the problem and that is environment.

Poor toilet facilities, foul smelling toilet and unfavourable surroundings, all contribute in a big way to the development of constipation. Above is a brief resume of some of the causes of constipation which account for a significant number of people who suffer from the malady. In addition, a number of organic diseases involving small and large intestines also produce constipation directly or indirectly. The list is quite big in this category but important ones are spastic colon, irritable bowel syndrome, diverticular disease, anal fissure, haemorrhoids, perianal abscess, hypothyroidism, carcinoma colon, etc. Since all this requires proper investigations and judicious opinion—a doctor is the best judge.

Management of Constipation

Management of constipation is not difficult, provided the person tries to understand his problem. What one wants to achieve is a good and regular bowel action accompanied with minimum conscious effort and discomfort.

First of all, the patient has to be talked about his food (type and quantity), bowel habits, emotional factors and environment. Often the question arises whether the person feels uncomfortable because of infrequent passage of small, hard stools or there is inadequate evacuation.

In the other category are people who suffer from symptoms of tiredness, headache and discomfort even after having a daily bowel action. In fact it is this factor which leads to a form of bowel neurosis and an obsession with it. The deep seated belief about regular bowel action and in its absence the ill effects of toxic products being absorbed may have to be dispelled from the patient's mind with assurance and patient explanations. In fact in some the feeling of incomplete emptying of the rectum may not be real.

The person who complains of constipation has to be taken into confidence. Reassurance and proper assessment of causes goes a long way in alleviating the problems. Toilet facilities must be improved both at home and at place of work. Person must cultivate the habit of early rising and going for walks both in the morning and evening.

One should not neglect to answer the call to nature, since it disturbs the normal adaptive mechanisms of the rectum. Lavatory seat must be adjusted and proper type of toilet provided. Avoid use of bed pan and preferably use a commode.

If a person does not get an urge even in the morning he may take a cup of tea or glass of water on rising and walk about. Generally it helps. Even otherwise, the habit of visiting toilet in the morning hours must be cultivated.

Late rising and the rush to go to work are important factors which have to be remedied. Similarly, emotional disturbances have to be adjusted. Some people who work in shifts may suffer chronically from constipation. If possible, change to regular hours be suggested. It must be stressed to the individual that there is nothing like once in 24 hours schedule. Missing an occasional bowel movement should not be source of unnecessary anxiety.

Diet

Most of the times the main problem lies in the faulty habits of eating like missing of meals or taking meals at irregular times or taking only soft foods. This factor must be corrected. Food should mainly consist of roughage, salads, fresh and green vegetables.

The diet must be robust one with generous supply of fruits, fresh vegetables like carrots, radishes, lettuce, spinach, whole wheat bread, oats, nuts, etc. Where person is accustomed to take soft foods, bulk forming substances like beans, cereals, china grass, agar-agar, bran, etc. may be added. Similarly, the person must take large quantities of fluids like fresh water, lemonade, fruit juices etc. Use of confectionary, pastries, sweetmeats, cakes, bananas be curtailed, since they are constipating foods.

Food rich in fibre includes whole grain, oats, whole wheat atta, unhusked rice, alfa-alfa and the best vegetable sources are leafy green vegetables, asparagus, celery, cabbage, cauliflower, lettuce, root vegetables like carrots, radishes, turnips, etc. Fruits like papaya, oranges, apples, melon, watermelon, guava be preferred.

In the Indian diet there is no problem of taking a high fibre diet and it is mainly improper advice about food habits as well as food fads of people which really creates problems. As a general rule the person who suffers from bowel dysfunction must ensure a robust diet containing plenty of fresh fruits, vegetables and fluids. Take enough fluids to keep the gut 'wet'. Cut on soft foods like pizzas, sweets, highly spiced and greasy food.

Laxatives

Most people use laxatives without properly understanding their action and this leads to a form of habit formation and a vicious circle. Used with care, they may help to some extent.

Strong purgatives are not desirable, since they result in loss of fluids and electrolytes from the body but a mild laxative given at a stage when the person starts complaining of constipation rather than waiting it to become fully developed, is more helpful and beneficial.

Then the question arises as to which type of laxative be given if it has to be. Ideally, a mild laxative should be employed. Laxatives which increase the bulk and thus supplement the insufficient dietary roughage are very useful, since they produce their effect by increase in bulk, holding small amounts of water and thus softening the faeces with resultant expulsion. In this category isabgol (Isogel) is very good and generally two to three teaspoonfuls either at bed time or in the early hours of morning are quite useful. Other laxatives in this category are agar-agar, the pulp of bael fruit, etc.

Liquid Paraffin

It is a soft lubricant. Its main action is confined to the lubrication of intestinal mucosa and thus helps the faecal matter to pass off smoothly.

On taking it orally, it has a tendency to enter the trachea with subsequent deposition in the lungs causing a serious health hazard, producing Lipoid pneumonia. This risk is more in small children, elderly and debilitated patients. Its main disadvantage is that it may seep through the anus and spoil the clothing. Similarly, its prolonged use interferes with the absorption of fat soluble Vitamins A, D and K. Usual dosage is 1 oz at bed time either plain or with milk.

It is recommended for cardiac patients, pregnant women and for very ill persons. It is especially useful when straining at bowel action is not desirable.

As a general rule only mild laxatives are recommended. Use of strong purgatives is now no longer advised, since they are irritants to the intestines and at the same time lead to loss of electrolytes and fluids from the body.

Magnesium Sulphate is a useful saline purgative and is used when a strong evacuation is desired.

Castor Oil is a strong purgative. It results in excessive loss of water, electrolytes and of unabsorbed nutrient material. Its use in pregnant women, ill persons and elderly people is contraindicated.

For general use very mild laxatives are to be used and these include dulcolax, senna, pursenid and milk of magnesia, etc. Sometimes especially in children rectal suppositories are also employed.

The smallest effective dose of a laxative should be used and gradually discontinued once the bowel movements become regular.

To sum up, one would appreciate that constipation is to be treated preferably by general measures and one should use laxatives only in early stages to help the bowel movements. Gradually with diet, exercise and regular toilet habits, one can get rid of the condition. Those people who become slaves to laxatives and purgatives can never come out of this problem and one vicious habit goes on leading to another with resultant ill effcets.

LAXATIVES — THEIR USES AND ABUSES

13

Constipation is universally prevalent. It is more a disease of civilization, since almost all the people who are tuned to modern day living have suffered and do suffer from constipation at sometime or the other in their lifetime.

But it is the habitual constipation which really creates problems for the person. Non-passage of a daily motion does not necessarily mean constipation. In fact a person suffers from constipation when his regular bowel rhythm is disturbed, the stools become dry and hard and there is sense of ill health and discomfort.

The norms of so-called values about bowel action differ from country to country and race to race. Thus an Indian patient may not be satisfied with the passage of one motion a day, while his counterpart in the West may be satisfied even with the moving of his bowels only two or three times a week. A number of factors may be responsible for the production of constipation. These range from faulty diet habits, leading a sedentary life, ignoring the call of nature, irregular bowel habits, dirty toilets, crowded living to disordered action of the muscles of the abdomen and colon. To a great number of people, there is an obsession with the number of bowel movements per day and often there is a feeling of inadequacy about either the amount of stools which may be too little or there is a sense of inadequate emptying of bowels.

Daily passage of faeces is not essentially the way of living in a great majority of people especially those who take soft diets. This is not constipation and does not call for the use of any drugs. A person suffers from constipation only when the irregularity of bowels causes a sense of ill-being and discomfort.

The management of constipation means an approach at varying levels which should strike at the very causes of it. Use of high residue diet, leading an active physical life and regulating one's bowel habits shall go a long way in correcting constipation. The person should be encouraged to take fibre-containing foods. Fruits and vegetables like apple, papaya, carrots, brinjal, cucumber, spinach, sarson ka sag and members of the cabbage family should form the main bulk of food. One should preferably avoid mangoes, bananas, sweets, cakes, pastries, puddings and chocolates, etc. Salads, orange juice, oat, meal porridge, whole wheat bread, fibrous vegetables and nuts should be other constituents of food.

A liberal use of fluids like mineral water, fruit juices and milk, etc. must be encouraged since adequate quantities of fluids in the abdomen shall prevent the stools from becoming dry and hard. Unfortunately, very few people realise that it is the properly regulated habits rather than purgatives or laxatives or aperients which shall correct the constipation.

Often a person avoids the urge to pass a motion and thus suppresses what is a natural phenomenon. Quite commonly such people may not pass a motion again for number of days and then a compulsive need to swallow a laxative may arise which gradually becomes a habit and it may be repeated ad lib.

An occasional use of a purgative or a laxative is well within normal norms but the sad part is that laxatives are more abused than used judiciously.

A purgative (L. Purgativus – Purifying) means purifying substance while laxative derived from Latin word Laxativus which means loosening. At the same time aperient (L. Aperiens) means one which opens up.

Purgatives, laxatives and aperients are labelled as cleaning agents, since they are considered to purify the body of its toxic products.

A great number of people use them regularly under the wrong belief that their regular use shall rid the body of its waste products. For such people there is probably a fixation complex that unless they take a salt aperient in the morning and pass two or three motions per day their body cannot be excreted of its toxic materials. To such people, taking of a laxative or health salt is more of an addiction rather than a necessity.

A large number of people suffer because of the long continued use of laxatives or purgatives. In fact an addiction develops with all its resultant drawbacks. The result is that such persons often complain of marked tiredness, since they are regularly loosing minerals and fluids from the body with resultant apathy and a sense of being unwell.

Regular use of laxatives leads to addiction which is not uncommon amongst people. The interesting part is that the person may complain of looseness of bowels and is rather secretive about the use of laxatives. He or she may not even give a history about the use of such drugs.

Laxatives are good substances if used judiciously and with discrimination. It is their indiscriminate use which interferes with the normal functioning of the intestines both small and large. Their long continued use gives rise to loss of electrolytes like sodium, potassium and lot of fluid from the body. Long term use of laxatives interestingly results in constipation, since now the intestines which were earlier on having their normal movements, get tuned to the use of a laxative and won't move till some artificial stimulant is used. Apparently laxatives should be used with care. One sane rule for taking a laxative is "Do not take so much that loose stools result and at the same time take enough so as to prevent recurrence of constipation."

Stact with food-take containing roughage along with adequate intake of fluids and physical exercise. Laxatives be taken as temporary measure. As soon as regular habits are achieved the dosage of laxatives should be reduced and then gradually withdrawn.

There are number of similar measures as compared to drugs which shall correct the constipation. Thus a stimulus to initiate defecation like small exercise on waking up like a walk, use of bed tea or a glass of water or nimbu pani are very good natural laxatives, since the presence of food or liquid in the stomach especially in the early hours of the morning helps in starting a reflex (gastrocolic) which may be sufficient stimulus to evacuate the intestines of faecal matter. In case of flabby muscles of the abdomen, small massage of abdomen to tone up the flabby muscles shall help. This massage should be done from right to left and along the course of the large gut. Apparently properly regulated habits combined with use of diet containing enough of roughage and fluids, regular meal hours and toilet habits rather than purgatives are going to correct the sluggish bowels. Laxatives have to be used only when one cannot help their use and that too very occasionally.

One of the sanest advice on the use of laxatives is that the smallest effective dose should be used and gradually reduced when the bowels become regular. This is clearly much more rational than the intermittent treatment with comparatively large doses.

Let us look at some of the commonly employed laxatives.

Liquid Paraffin

It is an oily substance and is one of the commonest used laxatives either in pure form or combination with other drugs in the form of proprietry medicines.

In moderate dosage and occasional use it is a harmless laxative but when used over long periods it interferes with the absorption of nutrients and fat soluble vitamins like A, D, E and K.

Seepage of the drug through anal canal may take place at night, thus spoiling the clothes which aesthetically is not a very desirable thing. Often itching round about the anus may result. A very serious hazard with its use is the deposition of the drug in lungs, resulting into a serious ailment called lipoid pneumonia. This is due to seepage of the liquid paraffin in lungs through the pharynx especially at night when the person is asleep. This danger is more so in small children and elderly persons.

In old persons this hazard is much more pronounced, since when they take it at bed time a small amount of it remains in the throat and mouth. As the cough reflex in these people are weak and less sensitive the result is aspiration of the oily liquid and over a period of time a considerable amount of oil accumulates in the lungs and produces inflammation. Similarly, prolonged use of liquid paraffin will subsequently result in its absorption in the body and deposition at various sites leading to the start of tumour like structures called "Paraffinomas". This is a serious condition and is irreversible despite the fact that a person may discontinue the use of the drug.

But an occasional use of liquid paraffin does not produce these harmful effects. It is only in those people who consume it in large quantities and over long periods that these deleterious effects occur.

Apparently there is strong advice about avoiding its habitual use.

Saline Laxatives

Of the commonly used, magnesium sulphate is the one most often employed. These laxatives act by means of their low absorbability, bulk producing action and the presence of large quantities of fluids in the gut which soften the stools.

It produces loss of fluid, disturbance of electrolytes and even interferes with the absorption of foodstuffs in the gut.

These have to be avoided in cases of kidney damage and those who suffer from heart failure.

Castor Oil is a very strong purgative and produces severe griping in the abdomen with resultant loose motions. Taken over long periods, it results in excessive loss of fluids and electrolytes from the body.

Phenolphthalein is a contact (stimulant) purgative. It is partly absorbed and re-excreted in bile. It is used in the form either alone or in combination with other preparations like paraffin (Agarol).

Except for the fact that its prolonged use may result in interference with glucose absorption very few side effects are known. Drug sensitivity reactions may occur and are quite common with it. It should be used with caution during the first three months of pregnancy. Along with laxative use of milk and antacids be avoided.

Dulcolax (Bisacodyl) is a comparatively mild laxative and has its main action on the large gut. It can be used in tablet form or suppository in case of children.

Prolonged use may result in severe abdominal cramps.

Stool Softners are a mixture of two or three drugs and have toxic effects on the upper gastrointestinal tract and biliary function.

Senna and its compounds like Pursennid (Calcium Sennosides) are probably safe stimulants of intestinal movements. In usual dosage they do not have any effect on water and electrolytes in the body. They are also not known to disturb the digestive functions of the intestines. Side effects include nausea, vomiting, skin rashes, drug eruptions, etc.

Though in the usual dosage these are safe and mild laxatives but their repeated use over long periods damages the intestinal mucosa and produces inflammation and pigmentation of the colonic mucosa (Melanosis coli).

Lactulose: It is a semi-synthetic disaccharide of fructose and lactose. It is not digested or absorbed in the small intestines. It is broken down in the large gut by bacteria to osmotically more active products. It is effective for people suffering from chronic or habitual constipation. Dose 15-30 ml two to three times a day. It should be used with care in pregnancy, children, diabetes, elderly and debilitated people.

Isabgol Husk: It is the simplest and safest purgative and is safe. Two to three teaspoonfuls taken at bedtime either with milk or water is the usual dose recommended. But only precaution is that it should not be swallowed dry as it may cause oesophageal impaction. People with pain in abdomen or distension should avoid it.

Taking the question of use of laxatives as a whole it is the long, continued use of any of these purgatives or laxatives which produces its harmful effects. There is loss of fluids, precious electrolytes and the person suffers from marked weakness of the body. Skin may loose its shine and they have what is called woe-begone or a haggard look.

In those who have been taking laxatives for very long periods irreversible damage to the large gut may occur. Such people have to be weaned away from the addiction gradually by the use of drugs, sympathetic advice and persuasion. In severe cases the loose motions become a constant feature even without the use of purgative. In the words of Sir Avery Jones, these addicts have "Purgation without purgatives and especially at risk are those who were subjected to ritual purgation when young and have continued the habit into adult life."

In addition to drugs, constipation is also treated by other means like the use of suppositories, soap and water or glycerine enemas. Repeated use of enemas has its own bad effects. There may be loss of fluids and electrolytes from the body. Damage to the mucosa of the large intestines may occur. Sometimes, the whole procedure may be very discomforting.

Use of laxatives or purgatives has its own hazards in elderly people and pregnant women. In elderly persons mild laxatives only should be used, since they are likely to suffer from disturbances of fluid and electrolytes. During pregnancy very few laxatives should be employed and in fact the use of purgatives is not only ill advised but also unnecessary. Liquid paraffin is considered safe but it also interferes with the absorption of nutrients. Strong purgatives are undesirable, since they not only upset digestive functions but also induce excessive intestinal movements because of their stimulant action on the gut.

One would appreciate that the use of laxatives has its own hazards. Weighing all the pros and cons, one would agree that majority of the cases of constipation can be cured without drugs if proper advice in the form of taking fresh vegetables, fruits, whole wheat bread, etc. is followed. One should lead a physically active life. Habit of regular bowel movements should be instituted at an early age. Meals should be taken at regular intervals and in proper manner. If one looks after the body, it shall take care of the bowels itself.

One should take course to laxatives or purgatives only as a last resort. In case you are a laxative addict then earlier you break the habit, better it shall be for your body and health. One must employ laxatives judiciously and not abuse them. If used judiciously laxatives are of good help to the disordered bowel functions but unfortunately they are not employed discreetly. So use laxatives only when you must and abandon them after achieving the regular bowel functions at the earliest. Always take recourse to healthy food habits and living and there is no reason why one has to become dependent on laxatives.

LOOSE BOWELS

14

The problem of constipation and loose bowels (Diarrhoea) is of common occurrence and involves alterations in the pattern of defecation habits. In fact in both there is deviation from the normal: while in former there is undue delay in the clearing of bowel, in the latter there is not only frequent passage of loose ill formed stools but also distressing symptoms of exhaustion, dehydration and general weakness. Diarrhoea or loose bowels is not a disease in itself but symptomatic of some other disease processes. Diarrhoea is a form of disturbance of intestines motility and absorption whichever and by whatever means initiated. It may become self perpetuating giving rise to marked disturbances in the body, resulting in frequent passage of liquid stools.

Loose bowels may be coming on suddenly in acute form or be chronic of some standing, may be in months or even years, defying management and causing lot of physical and mental agony to the sufferer.

All ages are susceptible to suffer from loose bowels and probably small children and infants are the greatest victims of the ailment which may look very simple and not very serious to start with. Diarrhoea in children is due to a number of causes and it is closely linked with the hygiene, sanitation and feeding habits of the child. As in adults it is only a symptom of a much serious ailment which is lurking somewhere in the body.

A number of factors contribute to the causation of loose bowels in young children. Thus diarrhoea is common in summer and rainy season, since this is the time when filth and flies are in abundance. Congested, over populated localities contribute in a long way towards further aggravating the disease process.

Appropriately diarrhoea in children occurring during summer months, has been called "Filth Diarrhoea." Very small children and infants fall an easy prey to the infection from the unclean feeding bottle and no doubt that it is now being advocated to breast feed the small child. Though there are numerous reasons to propagate this, yet one of the important reasons is that bottle fed children are likely to suffer more from loose bowels than the breast fed ones.

Surprisingly both over-feeding and under-feeding can cause loose bowels in children. Over-feeding is a well-known ill to which over indulgant mothers suffer from. The child is generally a male issue, probably the only one and the darling of the family. The result is that he is besieged with all type of delicacies and is encouraged to gorge them down. No doubt the result is indigestion, upset tummy and diarrhoea. The other example of children suffering from hunger diarrhoea is not difficult to imagine. Most of these children cry because of hunger and swallow lot of air. The intestines show excessive movements. There may be colic and the child passes green stools.

Similarly, the quality of food given to the child also influences the bowels. Too much of food whether carbohydrates, proteins, or fats shall result in looseness of bowel. Where a child is fed on large quantities of protein in diet, the stools are bulky, watery, foul smelling and yellowish green in colour, while those taking large amount of carbohdyrates have large amount of gas in abdomen accompanied by large loose stools with soreness and redness around the anal region.

But the biggest cause of morbidity in children is infective diarrhoea. In this the child passes large watery foul smelling stools which are yellowish green in colour. There is toxaemia and the child is ill-looking. There may be severe pain in abdomen. This group may be suffering from either bacillary or amoebic dysentery. In the former group the child may pass 20 to 30 stools a day which are small containing blood and mucus, while in the latter group the stools are large containing very little of faecal matter but lot of blood.

Many a small child suffering from acute infection somewhere in the body shows up with diarrhoea. Caution is necessary in such children, since these require treatment of body infection and not only of looseness of bowel.

Similarly, milestones like teething in small infants often gives rise to looseness of bowel. Again food allergy or milk allergy may manifest in the child with diarrhoea where loose watery foul smelling stools are passed.

But one thing is quite clear. A young child's intestines are uniquely sensitive to illness in other organ systems. An adult may suffer from severe infection but still not be having any looseness of bowels while a child may show up with loose bowels and vomiting even with a little infection in the ear. Infections by bacteria, viruses all give rise to diarrhoea and at times antibiotics prescribed for an infection in the body may provoke the looseness of bowel and often both the physician and the parents of the child are kept wondering as to how the child is still suffering from looseness of bowels when he/she is on strong antibiotics.

One must not ignore the fact that antibiotics and their indiscriminate use often kills the normal intestinal flora leading to diarrhoea. But every looseness of bowel in a child is not always acute. In most of the children what appeared to start as an acute process now tends to becomes chronic, causing lot of anxiety to the parents. A broad definition defines that if the loose and too frequent stools persist for more than a week in a child or infant, this diarrhoea should be labelled as chronic. Similarly, this chronic diarrhoea in children may not be of much significance and may settle spontaneously but in a number of cases it may portend the presence of a serious disease.

A number of conditions ranging from bacteria, parasites improperly digested food to malabsorption may account for it. There may be another group where despite all the elaborate investigations the diarrhoea does not fit into any specific group and this is what is called the idiopathic group. Most of such children are robust, active but do pass loose stools frequently and for long periods. In some, it is believed that they are suffering from the subclinical state of a chronic malabsorption while in others it is considered to be the continuation of an invasive enteritis. Often either there is a fungus infection or excessive use of drugs which could account for this diarrhoea.

In majority of cases of chronic diarrhoea in children there is persistence of infection due to bacterial pathogen or as a result of damage to the intestinal wall during the acute episode.

Of the parasites, round worms, thread worms and others are equally responsible for causing chronic diarrhoea. Giardia, a racket shaped parasite is an important cause of chronic diarrhoea in children. These children may sometimes suffer from acute symptoms but often they pass large foul smelling, frothy and mushy stools. Food and especially milk allergy is another important cause. Allergy to either cow's milk or food should be considered when there is association of diarrhoea with skin rashes. Removal of offending food from the diet makes the symptoms of diarrhoea disappear within two days.

Another commonly encountered feature is the presence of diarrhoea with undigested food in the stools. This child despite the diarrhoea has normal growth and development and this symptom complex goes by the name of irritable bowel. Most of these children are emotionally disturbed. Correction of the social and emotional factors in the child's surroundings both at school and home go a long way in improving their condition.

But then a number of other causes like diarrhoea following abdominal surgery, enzyme deficiency, coelic disease, pancreatic insufficiency due to fibrosis and malabsorption syndrome all can account for chronic looseness of bowel which may defy treatment on conventional lines. Most of such children pass loose, ill-formed pale, frothy and stinking, but not watery stools which are more bulky than the food taken. Such children waste and suffer from malnutrition. The wasting of body tissues is apparent more in the limbs than on the face. Such a child requires proper assessment and investigations. Apparently, diarrhoea in such cases is not a disease but a symptom of some more serious ailment. Similarly, diarrhoea in an adult to a large extent runs parallel to its picture in a child.

And it cannot be denied that diarrhoeal diseases are to a large extent responsible for worldwide morbidity and mortality. Directly or indirectly they take heavy toll of human life. One rough estimate puts that in any given 24 hour period 200 million people on earth have gastroenteritis, most commonly diarrhoea and that too most likely due to bacterial infections.

Gastroenteritis

Bacterial infections are important cause of acute diarrhoea. These include Shigella, E. coli, Salmonella and Staphylococcal infections and are characterised by profuse watery stools, lower abdominal cramps and pus and blood in stools. Most such diarrhoeas come acutely, generally following consumption of contaminated food or water. It has a short fulminating course, characterised by headache, chills and abdominal discomfort. There may be rise in temperature accompanied by nausea and vomiting.

The source of infection remains the reservoirs in man and animals. Food, milk and water become infected from contamination and infection may be carried by flies. This malady becomes more in summer months and in people who do not follow the elementary rules of hygiene. Susceptibility also increases in people with poor nutrition and those suffering from chronic debilitating illnesses.

A number of viral infections are equally associated with high incidence of acute diarrhoea and these include poliomyelitis, measles and influenza infections. Viruses especially of ECHO group and Rota viruses are known to cause epidemics and now viral dysentery has been considered to be more common than bacterial or protozoal diarrhoeas. Viral diarrhoea is often accompanied by headache, fever, sweating, anorexia and malaise. There may be shivering and chilliness. Stools are watery and rarely contain pus, blood or mucus.

Cholera

Another important cause of acute diarrhoea and associated with high morbidity and mortality occurring mostly in India and surrounding countries is cholera, which takes great toll of human life. The victims of this entity pass large watery, rice coloured stools, have vomiting and show marked collapse, prostration and muscular cramps.

Cholera is an awe-inspiring disease which runs so rapid a course that a man in good health at dawn may be dead and buried at dusk. The great Hindu physician Sushruta as early as 5th century wrote about a disease similar to cholera. A serious outbreak of cholera in Jessore (Bangladesh) in 1817 was probably the starting point of the first cholera pandemic in world. In fact Bengal has been considered as the home of cholera. Epidemics of cholera have occurred in times of war, famine and at times when there is large collection of people as at fairs, melas, etc. Though it is nearly eradicated from other countries of the world, yet it is now localised to Indo-Pakistan subcontinent which constitutes the main nucleus of the world's endemic cholera today. Cholera is transmitted mainly through either contaminated food, water or by flies. Source of infection is always the human cases who are either convalescing from the disease or have recovered from it. Any natural calamity like floods, famine or places where people congregate like fairs, and festivals are harbingers of the epidemics of cholera.

Some people are more susceptible as compared to others. Thus starvation, excessive exhaustion, poor health, alcoholism and use of excessive purgatives especially during epidemics make the person an easy victim to the entity.

The whole disease process develops in a period spread over few hours to few days. Onset is sudden with violent purging and vomiting. The stools are rice watery in character containing flakes of mucus. Diarrhoea is very severe and has no pain. This either accompanies or follows very severe vomiting. If this stage continues, the person soon becomes moribund with sunken eyes, hollow cheeks and cold skin. There is marked anxiety, extreme thirst and restlessness. Temperature becomes subnormal and features of collapse and shock develop. This is the most serious phase and if recovery does not take place, death may follow soon.

Food Poisoning

Next in our list of causes of acute diarrhoea is 'food poisoning' which is much more frequent than is generally supposed. Often there is history of the person taking food from a common source as in an institute or a community feast and large number of people fall ill at the same time. There are many examples of food poisoning which have mild symptoms but it is the more serious one which gets noticed.

It is not difficult to arrive at the conclusions that the diarrhoea in a particular person is due to food-poisoning since several people who took of a meal have either acute gastroenteritis or signs of toxaemia. The source of infection is generally a stale contaminated food. Even stored food which has not been kept under proper refrigeration will produce food-poisoning. This is more likely to occur with milk and its various combinations and non-vegetarian food like fish and meat, since such foods get rotten early without adequate storage and refrigeration.

Botulism is rather a fatal form of food-poisoning due to organism clostridium botulinum. Meats and vegetables which have been preserved incorrectly in tins generally harbor the organism. In such cases the tin is generally swollen up indicating the presence of toxins. Food in such cases shows alterations in colour, consistency, smell and taste. Most of the persons show up with symptoms of illness within 24 to 48 hours after taking the infected food. Vomiting is very common, followed by nausea, abdominal distension and cramps associated with diarrhoea. Gradually nervous system gets involved, the heart rate goes up and blood pressure falls, death may follow soon. Other organisms responsible for food poisoning may be Staphylococci, Streptococci and Clostridium Welchii, etc. All these have got the same mode of infection, i.e., contaminated food and are characterised by nausea, vomiting, abdominal cramps and looseness of bowels.

Apparently acute looseness of bowel follows infection from a pathogenic organism which gains access through contaminated food or water. Poor hygiene plays important contributory role in this regard.

Traveller's Diarrhoea

Traveller's diarrhoea is another bug bear which effects travellers all over the world but especially people travelling to Africa, Arabic, Latin American countries and tropics, they suffer from an acute diarrhoea which often incapacitates the person soon after his arrival in that country. There is repeated passage of watery loose stools without any blood in stools, abdominal colic or signs of general ill health. Traveller's diarrhoea is one which probably accounts due to change in environment and climatic conditions *vis-à-vis* acquired immunity in local population. Most of the victims of traveller's diarrhoea are probably suffering from infection with E. coli, Salmonella, Shigella and Protozoal infestations like amoebiasis, giardiasis, etc.

Amoebiasis

Probably one of the commonest causes of diarrhoea in our country is due to amoebiasis. Acute amoebic dysentery generally starts insidiously without much general symptoms, the sufferer passes three to four stools with pain and tenesmus in abdomen. In the more severe form there is acute diarroea with griping pain and frequent passage of motions containing blood and mucus. To start with, the stools may consist only of fluid, blood and mucus. The stools have a foul odour and the blood is dark coloured. Generally, there is no fever but some degree of nausea and vomiting. Often there is superadded infection when signs of toxaemia appear. In most cases amoebic dysentery can be diagnosed in the presence of tenesmus associated with diarrhoea.

Giardiasis

Giardia, a parasite of worldwide distribution is responsible for causing chronic diarrhoea in children and young adults. It has also been considered to be an important parasite responsible for traveller's diarrhoea, since travellers have been known to contract it in virtually every part of the world. Often the infection is contracted by drinking infected water. Though a great majority of people suffering from giardiasis have no symptoms, yet the most common complaints of pcoplc with giardiasis is either an acute or chronic diarrhoea which may alternate with constipation. The stools are loose or watery and contain mucus but no blood. These people may suffer from abdominal colic, nausea, loss of weight, flatulence and fatigue.

Chronic Diarrhoea

But compared to acute diarrhoea is the problem of chronic sufferers of diarrhoea which takes its own toll. A number of factors may be responsible for the perpetuation of chronicity of the symptom complex. In specific distinction to children, chronic diarrhoea in an adult means when it is of more than three months duration. Bacterial and parasitic factors are to a large extent responsible for producing chronic diarrhoea. Sufferers of chronic amoebic infection often complain of disturbed bowel functions and in great number there are periods of passing loose, ill-formed stools interspersed with constipation. Tubercular exteritis is another common cause of chronic diarrhoea.

Over indulgence in green vegetables, salads and fresh fruits may be an innocent way of suffering from chronic diarrhoea. There is another group of people who are addicted to regular use of laxatives and no doubt they suffer from a form of chronic excess movements of bowels. A large number of people suffer from chronic carbohydrate dyspepsia and most of these people have a feeling of discomfort in the lower part of abdomen. Large amount of gas collects in the abdomen and during night it passes lower down, increasing the discomfort and often resulting in loss of sleep, irritation of the mucous membrane of the intestines and passage of large quantities of gas and loose small stools.

Lactase deficiency may be acquired late in life. Most such people complain of abdominal discomfort, watery diarrhoea and cramps especially within a short time varying from a few minutes to hours after the ingestion of milk and milk products.

Milk intolerance is very common amongst the Indian population and one rough estimate puts that probably one out of every tenth Indian is experiencing milk intolerance. It is due to lactose intolerance as well as deficiency of disacchacide enzyme in intestines, the acuteness of the problem depending on the degree of lactose deficiency. Impressions about lactose intolerance being responsible for causing chronic diarrhoea are not difficult to make when the history is there.

People who suffer from milk intolerance improve after discontinuing it. Since milk allergy is due to one of its constituents proteins like casein, lactalumin or lactoglobulin and since out of these three only casein is heat resistant, so a boiled milk may be tolerated by those people who are only allergic to either lactalbumin or lactoglobulin.

But a very important cause of chronic diarrhoea in adults is malassimilation of food substances ranging from carbohydrates, proteins and fats either due to diseases of small intestines or that of pancreas and this is broadly defined as a malabsorption syndrome. In a great majority of such patients the frequency of stools is increased to 5-8 per day. The frequency is greater in those suffering from small bowel disorders. The stools are large, bulky, pale, greasy, frothy, foul smelling, float on water and are difficult to flush, since they tend to stick to the pan.

There is marked and progressive weight loss and a sense of fullness or heaviness of abdomen more marked after 1-2 hours of taking food. Abdominal distension, gurgling sounds and colicky pain are frequent. Since there are disturbances in the absorption of food there is anaemia, soreness of mouth and tongue, dry atrophic skin, loss of hair and oedema of feet. Subsequently osteomalacia and neuropathy develop, causing pain in the limbs.

A number of diseases are responsible for causing chronic diarrhoea in malabsorption syndrome and these include pancreatic diseases, enzyme deficiency in small intestines, adult coeliac disease, tropical sprue, blind loop syndrome, intestinal tuberculosis, Crohn's disease, massive resection of small intestines, giardiasis and X-ray irradiation of small intestines, etc.

Tropical sprue is one entity which requires further discussion since it occurs mainly in tropics but its etiology still remains unknown. It is not a single entity but a syndrome characterised by chronic diarrhoea and marked weight loss, wasting, etc. The disease has existed since long. In the ancient "Hindu Texts of Medicine Charaka Samhita" it was suggested that this disease was due to weakness of digestive fire leading to impaired assimilation of ingested food.

In the tropics local population suffers from it and as these people travel outside their country, patients of tropical sprue are also being seen at other places. People of all ages suffer from it though adults are more prone to get it. Exact cause is not known though infection has been suggested. Cases occur both sporadically and in epidemics. There is damage to the intestinal mucosa but the exact cause of damage is not known. It may be due to either a dietary toxin or results from nutritional deficiency.

Majority of people suffering from tropical sprue complain of morning diarrhoea, loss of appetite and abdominal distension. In addition, they have pallor, weakness, sore tongue, oedema of the legs and even night blindness. The stools are watery, to start with, and become less liquid with the passage of time. Abdominal distension appears. Loss of weight occurs but there is no abnormal pain. Since the diarrhoea persists, features of nutritional deficiency appear but in some remissions and relapses take place and diarrhoea tends to disappear. Diagnosis of tropical sprue is not difficult, since all patients suffering from chronic diarrhoea and malnutrition in tropics are considered to be suffering from tropical sprue.

Coelic disease is another disease in which there is either actual or potential clinical malabsorption of most of the nutrient foods. Along with it there is a very characteristic lesion of the mucosa of the small intestines and these people are sensitive to gluten of the cereals with the result that the diarrhoea improves promptly when certain gluten containing cereals are withdrawn from the diet of the sufferer.

People all over the world suffer from it, though it is less in some and more in other parts of the world. People of all ages fall victim to it but the disease first becomes apparent in small children when they start with the cereals and these persist throughout the childhood if it is not recognised. Often it may disappear completely or diminish by the time the person reaches adolescence. But then it reappears either in the third or fourth decade. In some people diagnosis of this entity may not be reached till old age. Most commonly, the sufferer has severe diarrhoea, weight loss and marked weakness. The stools may be watery or semiformed, frothy and have a peculiar foul, rancid smell. The large putty like stools are difficult to flush down. Since these stools contain high fat and gas they often float in water.

Cases of coeliac disease have marked fatigue, lassitude and suffer not only from anaemia but also marked weakness. The person gets emaciated, looses weight and the skin folds become loose. Oedema over the legs and feet may develop. Skin may bruise easily and bleed. Abdomen becomes protubrant. There may be tenderness in legs because of neuropathy.

But mere passage of frequent stools does not mean the end of the picture. Taking the whole spectrum of chronic diarrhoea one can appreciate that if the stools are thin and watery it means that it is due to small intestinal hurry, while stools from the large intestines are generally thick and well formed.

Irritable Bowel Syndrome

Emotions also control the intestinal movements to a large extent. Nervous diarrhoea occurs in highly strung individuals or as a result of some situation producing emotional strain and is characterised by the passage of loose stools after meals. It may be apparent or working subconsciously but it is a great source of annoyance and suffering to the individual. Similar to this is the picture of irritable bowel syndrome which has been called by some as a disease of civilization. As has been pointed out, this entity should be expected in a tense anxious patient who is apprehensive, meticulous, rigidly conscientious or is deeply introspective. There are other features of anxiety like sweating, cold hands, flushing, rapid heart rate and tremors, etc.

Colon spasm occurs in such nervous individuals at times of anxiety and stress. The bowel motility becomes disordered with increase in mucous secretions. The irritable bowel (colon neurosis, spastic colon, muco-membranous colitis) is more frequent in sedentary, over ambitious people and is further aggravated by the use of purgatives, salads and raw fruits. Most of the sufferers have an emotionally unstable personality, they suffer from abdominal discomfort, pain and tenderness in the lower part of abdomen and some may complain of constipation rather than diarrhoea. Associated symptoms of neuroses are present. Some of them have got a fixation complex about their bowels and are often depressed. There may be recurrent constipation, diarrhoea or flatulence often occurring intermittently between periods of normal bowel function. Passage of large amounts of clear mucus without pus or blood in the stools is quite specific of irritable bowel which is direct contrast to cases of either amoebic or ulcerative colitis where blood and mucus are passed in stools. So making an impression about a sufferer of irritable bowel is not difficult, provided one is patient with the person in unearthing his or her hidden conflicts.

Irritable bowel is rather a form of disorder which manifests itself either in chronic or recurrent fashion at times of stress and emotional strain. Any situation which calls for acute stress such as occurs in war, at the time of examinations or even conditions of marital discord, all call for a condition the bowels may react violently.

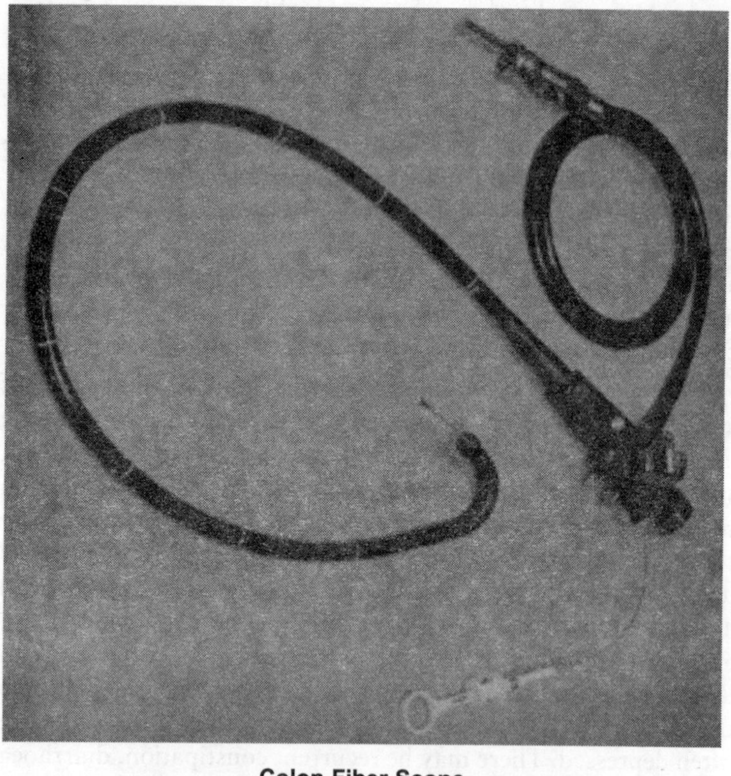

Colon Fiber Scope

The symptoms in most of the people are bizarre. There may be either a group of symptoms present singly or in combination with other symptoms. Abdominal pain may be present at times especially felt in the lower part of abdomen. It may be increased by the intake of either food or cold drinks. Passage of flatus or bowel movement gives some sort of relief.

Loose bowels are either constantly or intermittently present. The stools are loose, semi-solid, non fatty and may be small. There is great urgency. Often the person has to go to the bathroom immediately after taking food. Small amount of mucus may be present in stools.

The sufferer from irritable bowel goes to the toilet several times during the day, passing small quantities of soft or hard stools.

In addition to symptoms pertaining to bowels, these people often complain of excessive belching, loss of appetite, abdominal distension and mild nausea. There may be complaints of anxiety and nervousness in the form of palpitation, shortness of breath, sweating, flushing and headaches.

The characteristic personality of irritable bowel person is that of anxiety, aggression, tension and often depression. Hysterical traits are present in the personality. But most of such people are beset with problems of emotional tension and in these people the colon reacts in an abnormal manner. A number of factors like rapid ingestion of cold liquids or high carbohydrate foods, excessive use of condiments, spices and coffee may further worsen the condition.

It is not difficult to recognise cases of irritable bowel, since looseness of bowel in such people is associated with periods of stress and emotional tension of life.

An easy way of recognising such cases is that there is always temporary relief of pain associated with defecation. It always indicates that the colon is the culprit. Naturally the bowel habit in such people is variable. A number of foods in the diet like apples, pears, oranges, tomatoes, fresh salads, fried foods, milk, eggs, fish, coffee and beer may worsen or exacerbate the symptoms.

As far as psychological factors are concerned it is agreed that most of the sufferers from irritable bowel are over anxious and have a habit of constant worrying even bordering to the level of obsession.

Ulcerative Colitis

An important but serious cause of chronic diarrhoea may be ulcerative colitis which is an inflammatory disease of unknown and of multiple causes. It principally affects the rectum and lower part of left colon. It is a chronic disease characterised by remissions and relapses. There are loose bowels with blood and mucus. It appears in adult and early middle age most commonly affecting either in second, third or fourth decades. Often the patient ascribes the start of illness to an emotional trauma or some other alterations in life style.

The disease varies in its severity. The symptoms may range from the passage of small amounts of stools with rectal bleeding or there may be severe fulminant diarrhoea accompanied by considerable colonic bleeding, anaemia, weight loss, toxaemia and tachycardia.

Mild form of colitis is the most common form of disease and is present in 90 per cent of the people. Neither colonic bleeding nor diarrhoea is severe in such cases. Generalised symptoms of toxaemia are either absent or present very minimally. There is generally light bleeding in the absence of diarrhoea or there are short episodes of fatigue and lower abdominal discomfort. As the disease progresses the number of stools passed increases and these invariably contain blood. Mild low grade fever may appear. There are abdominal cramps, excessive fatigue and lack of inability to take interest in normal activities. But with severe form of colitis the whole disease process may progress to a critically dangerous point. These people have severe form of diarrhoea with excessive bleeding. There is moderate to high fever, features of toxaemia, abdominal cramps, tenesmus with frequent passage of bloody and watery stools. Patient looks very ill and is rapidly loosing weight.

So to look at the problem of looseness and increased frequency of passage of stools is not so simple and a layman is

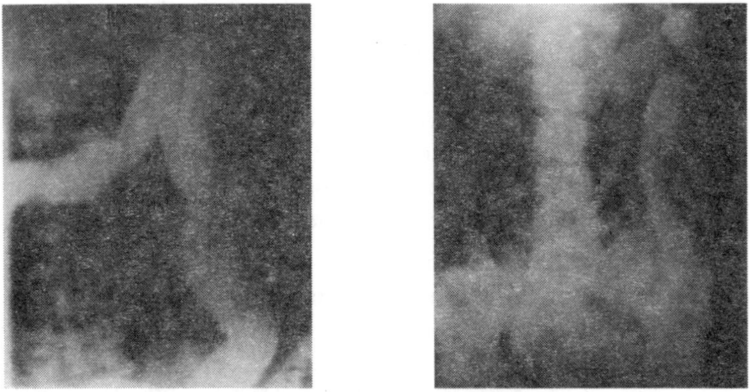

Barium Enema studies in case of Ulcerative Colitis

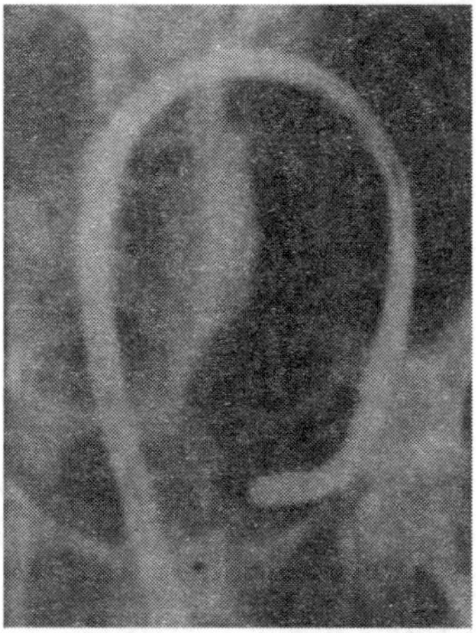

X-ray picture of abdomen with colonoscope inside

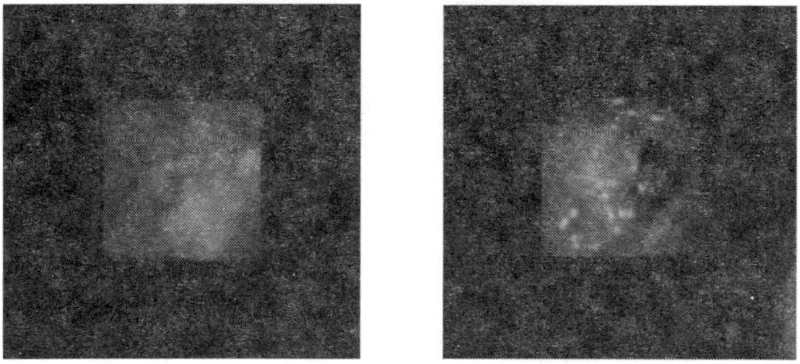

Case of ulcerative colitis seen through fiber scope

naturally worried when he or she suffers from it. Apparently one can evaluate the nature of illness in most of the cases, since acute diarrhoea is generally self-limiting and improves within a period of three to four days. One can also locate the probable site of the looseness of bowel depending on the character of the stools and the site, location and quality of pain in the abdomen. It is equally important to distinguish whether the diarrhoea is from the small or large intestines.

Diarrhoea of small bowel in origin will most likely be watery, loose, frothy, soupy or even greasy. It may contain undigested food particles and is free of blood. As compared to this the stools from large bowel are generally formed, thick, contain blood and mucus.

In diarrhoea of small bowel origin, there is urgency to pass small quantities of stools or in other words there is intestinal hurry. Similarly, in large bowel diarrhoea the faecal matter may be passed in any quantity, it may be mushy or even jelly like and is often mixed with mucus and blood. The passage of stools may be characterised by tenesmus and griping pain in the abdomen.

This is one clue towards arriving at the type of diarrhoea since it tells us as to the underlying factors whether the disease is in small intestines or large bowel. Similarly, a few points elicited about the looseness from the sufferer often points towards the real culprit. If there is history of diarrhoea following a party or ingestion of food from a common source, it is not difficult to conclude that diarrhoea in this case is infective. Similarly, food poisoning would be implicated when a number of people have fallen victims to it after a feast.

In children the source of infection may be traced to the bottle or diarrhoea coming at the time of teething may in fact be infection transmitted by the child's hands while playing in dirt. Diarrhoea following infection is generally sudden in onset and progresses or improves depending on the severity of infection. Looseness of bowel appearing from very childhood and then persisting on may be pointer towards its being coelic disease. History of allergy to certain foodstuffs like milk, soya shall underline the possibility of lactose intolerance or diarrhoea being of allergic in origin. Repeated attacks of diarrhoea accompanied by tenesmus shall be a pointer towards chronic amoebic infection while looseness developing after arriving at a hill station shall more likely go under the name of Hill or Traveller's diarrhoea.

When diarrhoea is associated with anaemia, malnourishment and defects in absorption of foodstuffs it shall probably be due to malabsorption syndrome. Similarly, emotional conflicts may be an indication that the person is most likely suffering from irritable bowel syndrome. A look at the stools, i.e., naked eye examination shall also tell a number of points which are helpful in arriving at some conclusions. Thus the presence of blood in stools indicates either an inflammatory or infectious process. Same is the case about the passage of pus or mucus in the stools. Lack of odor and presence of blood tinged mucus characterises stools of bacillary dysentery. Pea soup stools are characteristic of salmonella infection while rice water stools are typically seen in cases of cholera. Mushy, frothy, foul smelling, large, bulky stools which stick to the pan and are difficult to flush out are typically seen in cases of tropical sprue and malabsorption syndrome. Large formed stools containing blood and mucus shall suggest ulcerative colitis. These are just a few of the hints which may help the layman in reaching some of the conclusions about looseness of bowel but any looseness of bowel either acute or chronic has to be managed by a competent physician and investigations required especially in chronic cases.

Thus in every case stools (fresh specimen) are examined both by naked eye and under microscope. Stools cultures are indicated in cases of infective diarrhoea.

Examination of the patient along with a detailed family history, personal and social history also helps in arriving at some conclusions. In cases of irritable bowel or ulcerative colitis sigmoidoscopy/colonoscopy is undertaken to study the lower bowels for inflammation, ulcers, etc.

Radiological studies in the form of X-ray abdomen, barium study of small intestines and barium enema to study pattern in large intestines are undertaken.

Absorption studies like D-xylose test, faecal fat excretion, schilling test are undertaken to study the problem of malabsorption. Even colonic biopsies and jejunal biopsies are further done to help in establishing the diagnosis. But since these tests are better left to the care of the attending physician we shall now delve on the measures which may be undertaken to prevent suffering from looseness of bowel.

Most of the diarrhoeas in both children and adults are acute and at the same time infective in origin, so it is almost obligatory that if one has to escape from the morbidity of this illness, a minimum standard of hygiene must not only be enforced but also followed in daily life.

People who handle food must ensure proper washing of the hands with soap, etc. and this applies equally after going to the toilet. Any infection of the skin and hands must be treated promptly and the person barred from handling food till the infection is eradicated.

In places like festivals or fairs where there is big congregation of people, strict hygienic measures about food, water supply and disposal of excreta must be followed. Unripe/overripe fruit and food which is unprotected from flies must be destroyed and their sale banned.

A child's bottle must be properly washed and sterilised. Similarly, the child's hands must be washed and kept clean meticulously since in most of the cases the source of infection is generally from these places. Milk and its products must be properly pasteurized. Care should be taken not to use improperly stored food and especially meat, etc. which is not fresh or has not been stored properly.

A large number of cases of food-poisoning can be prevented if shops selling canned products keep a proper watch on these and do not sell any cans which show either dents or signs of corrosion.

In fact in most of the cases of acute diarrhoea both in children and adults the main source of infection is either the food handler who contaminates the food or it is basically the infected food which itself is either not properly cleaned, cooked or stored.

Water supply is equally important, since infective diarrhoea, cholera, amoebiasis and giardiasis, etc. may in fact be traced to it. It is desirable whenever the water supply is considered to be the source of infection, to drink water after boiling it for about 15 minutes. A number of other factors might be further elucidated in the management of chronic diarrhoeas.

Thus in cases of coeliac disease removal of gluten from the diet helps. Gluten containing foods like wheat, barley, oats, noodles, spaghetti are avoided and it helps the individual a lot. In fact special diets are made out for such people in a way that their diet remains well balanced and contains adequate amounts of fat, carbohydrates and proteins.

Tropical sprue or malabsorption specifically requires correction of malnutrition and anaemia. Cases with irritable bowel require special care about their emotional problems, and a great assurance about the benign nature of their illness. In many cases, anxiety is related to very trivial problems but the stress to the bowels is very severe. To such people generally the nature of the illness should be explained and they should be encouraged to understand the life situation and to meet them with proper challenge and fortitude. Attempts should be made to adjust their social and occupational life and in a great majority of people, success can be achieved.

Diet in cases of diarrhoea has an important role to play. In cases developing acute diarrhoea and who are not very ill it is better to stop all food for twenty four hours and put the person only on liquids like boiled water/light tea/ORS, etc.

As the condition improves fruit juices, soft boiled rice, khichri, moong dal or curd be taken. In acute stage milk should be avoided.

In chronic cases, proper attention be paid to give properly assimilable nutritive foods so that nutrition is maintained. Avoid salads, acidic foods, condiments, spices and fried fatty foods. Vegetables containing roughage and fruits which are hard to eat be avoided.

But looseness of bowels (Diarrhoea) involves a great physical and emotional strain in an individual. Chronicity of the disease process entails a great burden on the body's vitality and earlier the underlying disease process is treated better it shall be for the sufferer. But since treatment of diarrhoea and its accompanying medication requires skilful handling so a layman should leave it in the hands of his or her doctor and not indulge in self medication, lest the end results may prove more harmful.

15 SUMMER OR TRAVELLER'S DIARRHOEA

Come summer and there is exodus of families to hills for pleasure and relaxation. But number of times the pleasures of the trip are marred by a very common problem called the summer/hill or traveller's diarrhoea.

Correctly speaking, traveller's diarrhoea is one problem which effects travellers all over the world but especially people travelling to tropics who suffer from an acute diarrhoea which often incapacitates the person soon after his arrival in that place. There is repeated passage of watery loose stools without any blood in stools, abdominal colic/pain or signs of general ill health. This diarrhoea rightly labelled traveller's diarrhoea is probably due to change in environment and climatic conditions vis-à-vis acquired resistance which has developed in people of that place. But then some of these people who suffer from this type of diarrhoea are also probably suffering from infection with bacterial (Salmonella, Shigella, E. coli) and Protozoal infections like amoebiasis and giardiasis, etc. It is the change in the milieu of the person coupled with dietetic indiscretions which brings on the acute illness. Just like traveller's diarrhoea, hill diarrhoea is also a very common ailment from which holiday makers suffer during their visit to hills in summer months. Hill diarrhoea is confined to people in tropics. It occurs in people coming from planes who visit hill stations situated at 6000 ft or above. Though many physicians believe that the cause of this diarrhoea is not exactly known and number of factors have been accounted for, yet infection with pathogenic organisms cannot be ruled out. There may be change of flora in the intestines but some organisms may be grown from intestines itself. The sufferer from the ailment is uncomfortable. There is flatulance, abdominal distension and morning diarrhoea. The person passes stools urgently four or five times before noon and surprisingly after that he is comfortable. The stools are large, pale coloured, frothy and do not smell.

But one must not forget that bacterial infections are also important causes of diarrhoea when a person is travelling to outstation. This is quite natural, since many people do not take adequate precautions about their food and personal hygiene. Sufferers from bacterial diarrhoea have profuse watery stools, lower abdominal cramps and pass pus and blood in stools. Most such diarrhoeas come acutely following consumption of contaminated food or water. It has a short fulminating course characterised by headache, chills and abdominal discomfort. There may be rise in temperature accompanied by nausea and vomiting.

The source of infection remains the reservoirs in man and animals. Food, milk and water became infected from contamination and infection may be carried by flies. The malady naturally becomes more in these hot months when elementary rules of hygiene may not be followed.

Viral diarrheoa has equally high incidence during summer months and now viral dysentery has been considered to be more common than bacterial or protozoal diarrhoea. This type of diarrhoea is often accompanied by headache, fever, sweating, anorexia and malaise. There may be shivering and chilliness. Stools are watery, ill formed and rarely contain blood or mucus.

Then most of our population either suffers from chronic amoebiasis or pass cysts of amoeba in their stools without showing any symptoms. It is very common practice to find people, after travelling or visiting a place after holiday, come back complaining of indigestion, abdominal discomfort and loose motions. The problem here is the conveying of infection to the victim through infected water supply or that the infection has been conveyed through a cook or a servant who has served the food. It is not difficult to appreciate the unhygienic habits of people who serve or cook food in small wayside hotels/*dhabas* who are going to be source of infection. Most of the food handlers have the bad habit of unclean hands, dirty nails and often scratch round about the anus and take the same fingers to the food and thus transmit the disease to others. Naturally the cook, if he or she is a cyst passer, shall infect the other persons. Cooks or waiters by their injudicious habits convey the infection to their unsuspecting patrons.

The factors of personal hygiene also cannot be minimized. Many persons do not wash their hands properly after going to the toilet and some have long dirty nails which harbour the amoeba in their nail bed. No wonder such people are acting as source of infection not only to themselves but also to others.

The sufferer generally gets acute diarrhoea and passes voluminous foul swelling, bloody brownish stools. There is generally abominal pain (Tenesmus) and feeling of exhaustion.

But generally speaking, every person who travels or visits a hill station during summer months does not suffer from diarrhoea. Reasons are that some people are more susceptible as compared to others. Thus starvation, excessive exhaustion, poor health, alcoholism predispose people to suffer more from such diarrhoeas.

Question arises as to what precautions should be taken to avoid falling a victim to summer/traveller's diarrhoea. Cases of hill diarrhoea last only for a few days as the disease is self limiting and subsides of its own. But if the ailment causes severe degree of prostration, exhaustion and there is blood in stools one must suspect that it is not plain hill diarrhoea but that there is either bacterial or protozoal (amoebic) infection for which correct medication should be taken. As a general rule whenever you are travelling, you must follow certain norms and precautions then only you can avoid falling victim to acute diarrhoea.

1. Whenever you travel away from home always eat less than what you have appetite for. Do not overeat and always avoid getting indigestion. Avoid overfried, rich foods. Salads should be washed properly before eating.
2. Ensure clean and pure drinking-water supply. Preferably use water after boiling. If not available then mineral water be substituted.

3. Do not consume either raw or overripe fruits. They are very common causes of indigestion. When taking non-vegetarian dishes and milk preparations like cheese, etc. see that they are not stale. A very common cause of food poisoning and diarrhoea in travellers is consumption of improperly cooked and stale food.
4. Maintain proper hygiene and avoid raw and cut foods available at rehris and in the market.
5. Do not travel on any empty stomach. If you travel with an empty stomach you are likely to fall victim to infection, since your body resistance is going to be low.
6. Take regular but light meals when you are outside your home at a holiday resort or in a hill.
7. Do not skip breakfast. A simple but adequate breakfast is essential for maintaining energy and protection against infection. Hungry stomach is as dangerous as overfull stomach.
8. Avoid excess consumption of beverages. Preferably do not take alcoholic beverages.
9. Preferably do not consume tinned foods or fruits. At many places these may be time expiry or old ones and there is danger of developing food-poisoning (Boutulism) which may sometimes prove dangerous.
10. Golden rules at a visit to hill camp/resort are: light, easily digestible food. Clean boiled or mineral water. Avoid cut, overripe or raw fruits and vegetables. Do not exhaust yourself. Take adequate rest in between your excursions. Always take lemon in your diet daily during your stay outside. But still if you fall victim to diarrhoea while at any hill station, etc. then
    - (i) First consult the doctor to find out the cause of diarrhoea and take proper medication.
    - (ii) Take plenty of fluids. Whey water, boiled water, light tea be preferred. Avoid getting dehydrated.
    - (iii) Take adequate bed rest. Do not get exhausted. Over exertion be avoided.

(iv) As you start improving, add semisolid foods like rice, khichri, curd, bread, boiled vegetables in the diet coupled with plenty of fluids.

With adequate care and precautions, there is no reason why your holiday should not remain an enjoyable trip.

16 DO YOU SUFFER FROM AMOEBIASIS

A widely prevalent disease and one of the most commonly encountered diseases in our country, Amoebiasis is of worldwide distribution. It is especially common in the tropics and hardly anybody escapes from it. Its victims present with a wide variety of symptoms, some odd, some common.

A disease of unhygienic habits, insanitary conditions and bad toilet habits, amoebiasis can occur anywhere in the world, since it is a cosmopolitan paratisite of man but it is the tropics and subtropical regions where the general poor standard of hygiene attracts the growth of the parasite and innumerable people are a victim to it.

A rough estimate places more than 500 million people throughout the world suffering from it. It is a disease of the tropics and subtropics, people in the temperate climates rarely having any symptoms. One estimate shows that probably more than 90 per cent of our population in India suffers from amoeobiasis in one form or the other, though various surveys have put its incidence in the various parts of the world from five to 47 per cent.

In certain closed communities like mental institutions, prisons etc. where ordinary sanitary measures are not up to the mark, a higher incidence shall be found. Apparently the incidence depends on various factors like socio-economic standards, hygiene and sanitary environments. Poorer the conditions worse the incidence. In our country almost every other person has either suffered or is suffering from amoebiasis. Since the disease runs in families, all the members of the family may be effected at the same time. Both the sexes are equally affected and no age has got any immunity. Even very small children are known to have been effected by the disease but as a rule it is generally the adults and young individuals who fall easy prey to it.

But what is amoebiasis? If you harbour the small unicellular organism called Entamoeba histolytica within you and whether you have any symptoms or not, it still means you suffer from amoebiasis. The organism gains entrance into the body via the mouth either in drinking water or food which is contaminated. Flies may directly or indirectly convey the infection.

The life cycle of the amoeba consists of three successive stages—Trophozoite (the growing or feeding stage), pre-cyst and cyst.

The trophozsite or vegetative form is the stage when the organism is exhibiting active movements varying its shape and is seen in the freshly evacuated dysenteric stools where it may be "giant sized." In contrast, it may be very small in the stools of a person who is having no symptoms. These amoebae live and multiply for a time in the large inestines living on the mucous secretions for their food. In the trophozite stage it is not infective and has no role in transmission of the disease but the danger here is more to the person who harbours the parasite, since it has properties of invading the tissuess. Subsequently the organism becomes quiescent, the trophozoites discharge undigested food and condense to form a special mass surrounded by a relative thin tough wall. This is the pre-cystic stage.

It is the cystic form of amoeba which is most important. Here the organism is spherical in shape surrounded by a membrane called the 'cyst wall'. A mature cyst has spheroidal body containing four nuclei and chromidial bodies.

The cyst is the infective and inactive stage which is found both in the large intestines as well as outside the body. It contains properties of resistance to the surroundings and can live for 10 days outside the body in suitable media like moist stools. It is destroyed by dessication (lack of moisture) and in temperatures above 50°C or below -5°C. These cysts are not destroyed by chlorination in the amount in which it is normally used for water purification. Boiling kills the organism.

Life Cycle of Entamoeba Histolytica

A large number of people pass the cysts of entamoeba in their stools without showing any symptoms. These carriers transmit the infection either by infected food, water, by their infected hands and nails especially if they are food handlers. Flies and cockroaches play important role in their transmission. Thus it has been rightly said that the oral route infection justifiably brings the factors of 'faeces' finger, flies, food and fluids' in the perpetuation of the disease.

Once the cyst is taken into the mouth and swallowed it reaches the stomach. The cyst wall is resistant to acid and so no change occurs. But as it reaches the small intestines it is acted

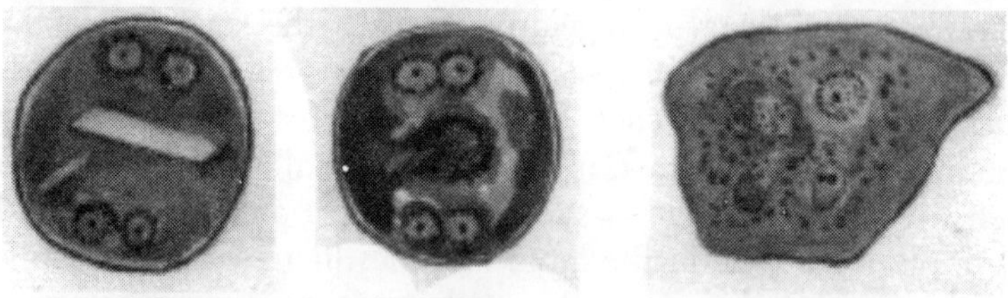

(a) **Cysts of entamoeba histolytica (Saline preparation)**

(b) **Iodine preparations**

(c) **Trophozite (active) form of E. Histolytica**

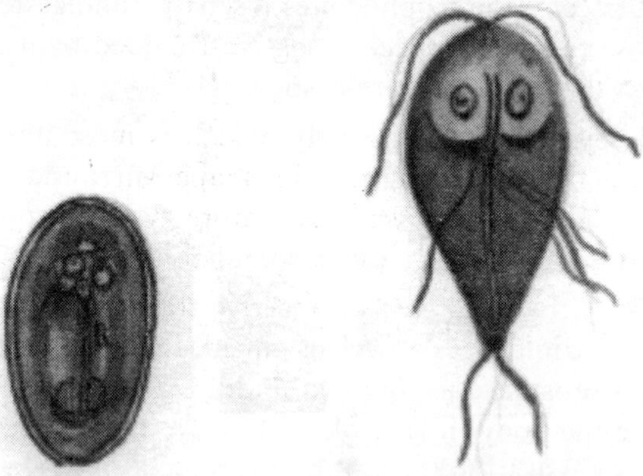

(a) Cysts

(b) Active (vegetative) form

Giardia Intestinalis

Cysts of E. Histolytica and Giardia

upon by the alkaline juices secreted by the pancreas, the imprisoned amoeba becomes active, escapes through a small rent and reaches the lower part of the small or large intestines. It is this stage when the organism is actively motile, has tissue invading properties, contains ingested red blood cells and as further development takes place, the amoeba now encysts. The earlier amoeba which had four nuclei subdivides and by further division of nuclei, eight amoebulae result. The end result is that out of every single cyst swallowed, there emerge not less than eight cysts.

Pathology

Once a person gets infected by amoebiasis the time taken to develop the symptoms of disease is variable. Generally, it is from two or twelve weeks. There are persons who have never had any attack of dysentery but still go on passing the cysts while in other category are logically those people who had an attack of infection, were not properly treated and now are a source of infection in the community.

Why some people, though severely infected, do not develop the disease is one of the poorly understood problems? The factor of poor nutrition, low protein, high carbohydrate diet, alcoholism have all been blamed as responsible for making a person harbouring the infection to fall easy prey to amoebiasis.

After the cysts have reached the large gut they mutliply actively, enter the wall of the gut through crypts reaching the submucosa. They secrete an enzyme and produce necrosis of the mucosa, shedding with it dead and necrotic mucosa, resulting into the formation of amoebic ulcers in the gut. Similar ulcers are produced through the length and breadth of the large gut which may become thickened and scarred sometimes having a flea bitten appearance; the ulcers varying in size from a pin's head to about an inch in size. The amoebic ulcer has a ragged edge and contains yellowish brown necrotic material. It may progress further invading the bowel wall and rarely perforation may result.

The parasite itself may work its way through the portal vein and be carried to other vital organs like liver, brain, lungs, heart, etc. resulting in the production of either inflammation or abscess formation. Liver involvement occurs very commonly with amoebiasis and either hepatitis or abscess is formed in the liver. In fact hardly any organ in the body escapes the brunt of the parasite. Rarely amoebiasis of skin, spleen, urogenital tract and of meninges results.

But what are the factors which predispose persons to get either intestinal or extra-intestinal amoebiasis?

It has been found that the bacterial flora in the intestines is very essential to the growth of amoeba and this indirectly influences the pathogenecity of the organism.

In addition, factors of virulence of the amoeba, low and poor resistance, poor nutrition, poor socio-economic status and addiction to alcohol are other factors which help in the propagation of the parasite at various sites in the body.

Predisposing Causes

A number of factors ranging from age, diet, climate, socio-economic status to personal hygiene habits have a significant role to play in predisposing a person to suffer from amoebiasis and its aftermath. Let us examine some of these factors.

Age, Sex, Race

No age, sex or race escapes amoeba. People of all ages and of races are affected. Very young infants apparently escape infection and understandably so.

Maximum incidences of the disease are found in people between the age of twenty and thirty.

Again the disease shall manifest more in the summer months and in a more serious manner, since it is the time when flies population is on the increase and general standard of hygiene is at a comparatively low level.

Diet

Most of the people who suffer from amoebiasis have got poor nutrition. Their diet is either mainly comprised of carbohydrates, hot chillies and spicy food or alcohol forms an important part of their food. Protein food is lacking from the diet. One opinion is that probably high protein diet kills the parasite-while the low protein diet tends to make the disease have a more flourishing course.

Climate

Hot humid climate is very good for the propagation of amoebiasis and that is why it is not only more rampant but also more severe in summer months in the tropics and subtropical regions.

Socio-economic Standards

Poor socio-economic standards indirectly determine the living standard and habits of the individual and his/her family. Lack of education not only general but specifically personal hygiene as well as regarding food handling, is an important reason why the disease is more prevalent among those with poor standards of living and hygiene.

The toilet habits of great majority of people leave much to be desired. Most of the poorer sections of society do not have proper latrines in their homes and even those who have they also do not observe proper sets of rules. It is a common site to see people defecating on the road side, in the fields and near water reservoirs like ponds, canals, rivers, etc. This results in infection of water which, when used for irrigation of fields, leads to the infection of vegetables which, when eaten raw, result in infection. Similarly, practice of using human waste as manure in fields further perpetuates the infection.

Water is also a great source of infection. When water is drunk from well, canals or for that purpose hand pumps, infection is likely to occur. Once water is infected ordinary chlorination does not destroy the amoeba and for that reason the ordinary tap water in the homes may be a source of disease.

Flies and cockroaches are other important source of conveying infection from infected stools to the food and water. But the most important place in this whole drama goes to the personal hygiene not only of self but of the cook in the house.

Most of the food handlers have the bad habit of having unclean hands and dirty nails. Some scratch round about the anus and take the same fingers to the food and thus transmit the disease to others. Naturally the cook, if he or she is a cyst passer, will infect the other members of the family. This is equally true of public places like hotels and hostels where the cooks or waiters may be harbouring the parasite and by injudicious cleaning habits convey the infection to their unsuspecting patrons.

Since hygiene in the family is interrelated so it is no wonder to find the whole family being the victim to amoebiasis. Naturally the familial incidence shall depend also on the common water supply, bad toilet habits of most of the family members and the cook (either the mother or the ayah or the servant) may be a chronic cyst carrier and infecting the food.

Symptoms

A large number of people suffering from amoebiasis may be just silent carriers of the parasite having no symptoms themselves but are just infecting the community. These chronic carriers are a dangerous lot as far as social hygiene is concerned.

The symptoms in majority of people are varied depending on the degree and virulence of infestation. Mostly the symptoms are either mild or ill defined.

Occasionally, when the trophozoites are active, the person gets acute dysentery with fever, pain, griping and repeated evacuation of voluminous, foul smelling, bloody brownish mucus containing stools. In chronic cases the person gets periodic attacks of diarrhoea alternating with long symptom free periods when there may be constipation.

Symptoms like dyspepsia, flatulence, nausea, heartburn and occasional loose motion with a feeling of ill health are quite common. A few may complain only of chronic constipation. Above are the people who suffer from chronic amoebiasis and are regular passers of cysts. Most of the times in such people the complaints are vague and ill defined.

Some people have a tendency to go to the toilet soon after taking any food while others have a form of windy abdomen or ulcer like dyspepsia. Appetite may be good in some, while in others it is lost or decreased. But it is the involvement of other organs besides the gut which requires more urgent consideration. Once the liver gets involved the patient experiences a sense of heaviness and discomfort in the lower part of right side of the chest and the upper part of abdomen. Fever generally of low grade appears and subsequently may even go up. There is rise in pulse and heart rate. Signs of toxaemia appear and because of the inflammation of liver there is not only dragging sensation but also pain varying in intensity from moderate to severe type. Liver is enlarged, soft, smooth and tender. Movements of the diaphragm on right side are restricted.

If not treated at this stage, the stage of hepatitis goes into abscess formation. Abscess in the liver may be single or multiple. As the abscess becomes bigger, toxaemia worsens. The patient becomes very ill, apathetic and emaciated. There is excessive sweating, tongue is furred. The patient complains of pain in the right side of abdomen while coughing. If still the abscess in liver is not treated it may burst either into the abdominal cavity or lungs, pleura and even heart resulting into death.

But most of the time the symptoms of liver involvement are very vague. Very occasionally history of having had acute diarrhoea in the past is not available and even if it is there, there may be an interval spread not only over weeks or months but even over the years. Normally the patient often forgets about it and ignores the symptoms. Besides liver, other organs commonly involved due to amoebiasis include abscess formation in lungs, brain, spleen, heart and genitourinary tracts. Lungs and heart may be involved either by direct spread or as a complication secondary to that of liver abscess.

Involvement of skin and meninges is not very common. Gut complications include haemorrhage, perforation and peritonitis.

Diagnosis

It is not difficult for a physician to make a diagnosis of amoebic infection in any person.

Stools examination is the sheet anchor in reaching the diagnosis. Stools for examination must be examined warm and as early as possible after passing. If examination is negative the fresh stools must be examined 5-6 times, since cysts are passed in cyclic fashion and a single examination may not be helpful. Again the person may use a saline purgative but not liquid paraffin or castor oil. Results become fallacious if the stools specimen is contaminated with urine or the person has been using antibiotics, bismuth, barium or charcoal for several days before collecting stool specimen for examination.

Stools are examined direct under the microscope with saline, iodine and eosin solutions. In some laboratories cultures of entamoeba histolytica are employed as a routine procedure. Serological tests (like complement fixation test, precipitation test, immobilisation test and indirect test) are mainly useful in diagnosing extra-intestinal amoebaisis, i.e., of the liver, lungs and other organs.

Other tests employed include radiology of the chest, abdomen, liver scan and aspiration of the liver abscess by needle.

Treatment

One physician wrote 'Amoebiasis is the regular resort of the diagnostic destitutes' but this is true to a greater extent, since amoebiasis is overdiagnosed in our country. Luckily, the therapeutic advances in its management have brought forth much greater alleviation in the sufferings of people.

Often the question arises that if on a routine examination of the stools amoebic cysts are seen should the patient be treated or not especially if he has no symptoms? The answer is 'yes'. The person must be treated because you never know when the disease may erupt into action.

A number of therapeutic agents ranging from hydroxyquinolones, furazolidine, furoxone, metronidazole, ornidazole, tinidazole and secondazole are available and effectively employed in treating the condition. Self medication by antiamoebic drugs is not advocated, since some of them are potentially toxic. There are reports of disease called subacute myelopathic opticoneuropathy (SMON) occurring in Japan and other countries of the region including India where prolonged use of antiamoebic drug Di-iodohydroxyquin (diodoquin, enterovioform) has resulted in blindness. Once the person complains of neuropathy and giddiness, the drug must be stopped but the disease is not completely reversible and some damage persists. This drug is now banned.

So treatment of amoebiasis must be done under medical advice.

Prevention and Control

Despite innumerable drugs available, the patient may not still be cured since the treatment of amoebiasis depends not only on drugs but also on a number of factors ranging from clean water supply to personal hygiene, good sanitation and proper surroundings.

Water is an important vehicle for transmission of cysts. Since faecal contamination is the main mechanism of transmission of the disease, infection naturally will be more where proper basic precautions about faecal contamination of water are lacking.

Apparently the bad habit of defecating in common places, roadside and fields, lack of clean water supply and defective hygiene are important bugbears for the perpetuation of disease in slums and rural areas. So the management, treatment and eradication of amoebiasis enjoins that

1. cultivate clean personal habits.
2. ensure proper disposal of human excreta.
3. clean and pure water be used for drinking.
4. wash all vegetables and fruits thoroughly before cooking and eating raw.
5. Protect food against flies and cockroaches
6. If you have a servant in your house, get him/her periodically examined for amoebiasis.
7. Proper training of toilet hygiene not only of the servant but of the whole family must be ensured. The hands must be washed thoroughly with soap and no dirt or faecal matter be allowed to be collected under the nails. Nails of the cook must be trimmed short.
8. Ensure general cleanliness in the surroundings and at least have a certain minimum standards of community and personal hygiene.

To conclude, one can say that though amoebiasis is of world-wide prevalence and the magnitude of problem is enormous and although a number of potent therapeutic agents are available, yet it defies eradication, since this is closely interlinked with general sanitation, insanitary conditions, over crowding, poverty and protein mlanutrition vis-à-vis personal hygiene and proper toilet habits.

17

DO YOU SUFFER FROM PILES

One of the commonest ailments suffered by the modern man which is very much connected with his living and habits is the development of piles which, in medical Jargon, is called 'haemorrhoids'. One rough estimate puts that by the time you reach middle age or cross fifties, more than fifty per cent of the people have fallen victim to this entity. It is equally, common in both sexes. Women fall victim to the disease as commonly as men.

Haemorrhoids are nothing but veins at the lower end of anal canal and they may be either internal or external. Both groups of vessels anastomose with each other freely so that bleeding occurs commonly from both the sources.

A number of factors ranging from heredity, occupation, chronic constipation, straining at stools to portal obstruction have been considered important causative factors.

Piles is another example of diseases of civilization. Modern man in its endeavour to go soft has discarded hard fibre containing foods, assumed sedentary habits and suffers from lack of physical effort. Since these people who take soft foods suffer from chronic constipation, they have to strain at the time of defecation and the effect of these efforts made to evacuate the hard pellets from the rectum is not difficult to visualise. Excessive straining induces a form of pressure on these veins which contain no valves and pressure associated with the erect posture adopted by the humans results in further strain and subsequent bleeding from these sites.

The effect of heredity in the development of piles cannot be minimized. It is quite common to see members of same family suffering from the disease. There is enough supportive evidence to show that persons who inherit poor supportive tissues are likely to fall an easy prey to the development of piles.

Any condition which increase the pressure in the abdomen either temporarily or permanently will predispose to the development of piles. Thus in pregnancy the woman is likely to develop piles in response to pressure from the pregnant uterus.

Lack of physical exercise and leading a sedentary life is another important predisposing factor. People who sit for long hours on chairs develop laxness of their pelvic muscles with the result that anchoring action on the vessels is gone, leading to increase in their tortuousity.

Occupations especially the ones which entail sitting at one place for long periods like office work, shop keeping and business, all entail sitting crouched up at one place for long hours without sufficient opportunity for exercise and leading of active life. In fact sedentary occupations have easier predisposition to the development of piles. But it does not in any way rule out the immunity of people who lead active physical lives from developing piles. It has been found that piles are found as commonly in sedentary indolent people than in physically active persons, though the incidence is definitely more in the former than in the latter. It only means that in physically active people some other factor operates.

Any other condition which increases the pressure in the portal venous system would contribute to the development of haemorrhoids.

Thus in women during the last three months of pregnancy progressively increasing pressure is exerted on the iliac vessels, which causes increased venous pressure in all the branches, thus affecting entire haemorrhoidal plexus. This is said to be a very likely situation for developing piles especially if the underlying factors predisposing to its development are already present.

Similarly, during labour, tension within the haemorrhoidal vessels increases and in those women who are fat and have already developed haemorrhoids or have tendency towards it, there might be acute bleeding immediately following delivery of the child. Here mechanical factors of stress on the vessels during pregnancy and delivery play an important role. Another theory has put the principal cause of piles as anal infection.

Posture of man has an important role to play. Man assumes an erect posture and there are no valves in his veins so that blood flows freely and there is no restriction to its free flow.

Infection makes a virulent attack on the venous channel comprising haemorrhoidal plexus. There is inflammation of the vessels with subsequent thinning and dilatation of the involved portions of haemorrhoidal vessels resulting into haemorrhoids.

In sum total, of all the causative factors responsible in the causation of piles, infection is now being given quite a high place. People of both sexes are involved, though the incidence of malady is less in people below the age of thirty and it goes up as the age advances.

Piles are classified into internal and external, depending on their position at the point of origin. Most of the sufferers from piles come complaining of passage of bright red coloured blood which may come either in streaks or in the form of a line along

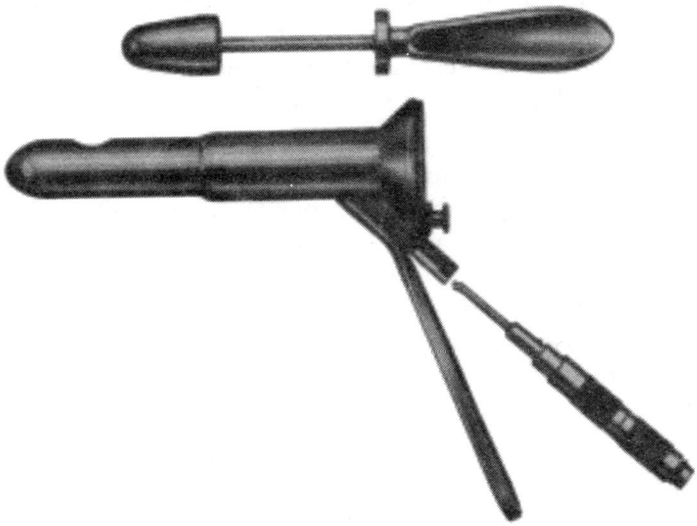

Proctoscope

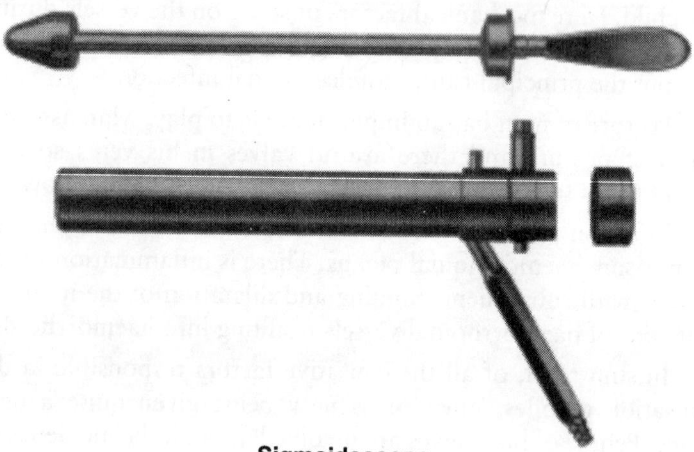

Sigmoidoscope

with the hard stools. Later on, it may spurt especially when the person is straining or may drip from the anal canal. Loss of blood and its appearance generally frightens the individual. Most of the chronic sufferers are victims of chronic blood deficiency and anaemia.

Bleeding in most cases of piles is from internal piles and is generally painless. It is usually bright red, unmixed with the stool, may occur before, in the course of or after defecation and may be expelled in large or small quantities.

When pain occurs it generally arises due to the involvement of one or more parts of all of the external haemorrhoids by acute inflammation. In the absence of infection and inflammation there is no pain. The pain shall be directly proportional to the amount of tension in the skin surrounding anal skin. It may be dull aching type increased by running, walking and hard labour. As the disease process becomes chronic, the pain tends to disappear. So the presence of pain in any case of piles means that the process has become acute.

As a general principle, external piles present no difficulty. One or more external piles may become engorged when straining at stools.

In some cases a bunch of vessels may protrude out of the anal canal like worms. This is called prolapse and often is accentuated when the patient coughs, sneezes or strains. The prolapsed tissue can be reduced manually in the beginning but subsequently it becomes irreducible. All this does not involve any pain and that is why most of the sufferers ignore the disease for a long time. When piles become infected pain and fever ensues.

A thrombosed external pile may be the individual's first experience with piles. Generally, it follows after an attack of acute diarrhoea or after a strong purgative or after the passage of a hard stool.

Piles depending on the degree of their involvement have been classified into first, second and third degrees.

First degree piles are mild and only protrude into the anus while second degree piles prolapse only to the extent that they can be reduced spontaneously. It is the third degree which creates problems and becomes so big that it has to be reduced manually. There is still another stage called the fourth piles which are almost irreducible.

Internal piles in their normal course are not visible from outside as compared to the external ones which can be seen by naked eye. So for looking at internal piles one has to take the help of instrument called proctoscope when they may be seen as somewhat accentuated or engorged vessels shining through the velvety rectal mucous membrane.

Once a person develops piles he or she must get it treated.

Patients in whom piles produce no symptoms may require no treatment but it is the person with symptoms who should be treated.

Piles management means both general and local measures.

General measures mean change in dietetic habits and living conditions. The individual must ensure adequate intake of fresh vegetables, fruits and salads in adequate quantities. Too much straining at the time of defecation must be avoided.

The person must respond to the urge to defecate as promptly as possible and to avoid sitting for long periods over the commode.

Active outdoor life coupled with participation in sport activities must be encouraged. Perineal exercises be done to improve the tone of the muscles of the pelvis.

Constipation and hard stools must be avoided. Stools may be softened and their passage eased out by the use of mild purgative at bed time. Infection round about anus and rectum must be treated adequately. Similarly, in all persons who show predispostion to haemorrhoids attacks of acute infective diarrhoea or amoebie infection must be adequately treated.

In a mild case of piles (Ist degree) generally relief is obtained by ensuring passage of soft stools, avoiding of constipation and of hard stools coupled with adequate perineal exercises. In majority of the cases relief is obtained.

But when supportive and palliative measures fail injection therapy is undertaken when a sclerosing liquid is injected into the tissues which surround and support a group of internal haemorrhoids. As a result of chemical irritation, the tissue shrinks and this shrinkage due to inflammatory reaction obliterates the haemorrhoids to varying degree. This is quite a safe procedure and success is achieved in great majority of people.

Injection treatment is not advised for external piles nor it is given when there is acute inflammation round about the rectum or there is any anal fissure or fistula. Similarly, injection treatment is not indicated for bleeding piles during pregnancy or in cases who have rise in pressure of liver (portal hypertension).

When injection treatment fails, surgical measures are adopted (Hemorrhoidectomy), i.e., the removal of haemorrhoidal tissue is the commonly accepted method. It may mean removing all external and internal haemorrhoidal tissue as well as obliteration of all routes of entry involved in the process of anal infection.

Main indications for surgery in piles are:

(i) Repeated attacks of disabling pain

(ii) Chronic bleeding, resulting in severe anaemia

(iii) Prolapse of haemorrhoids

And lastly, the most important one is the failure of palliative and injection treatment.

To sum up, an individual may be predisposed to suffer from piles not because of one factor but a number of factors ranging from hereditary predisposition, obesity, body built, sedentary habits, lack of physical activity, dietary habits, excessive use of soft foods, chronic constipation and factors which contribute towards increase in abdominal pressure.

Apparently a great majority of these factors are preventable and adequate precautions taken shall go a long way in preventing the person from suffering long-term deleterious effects of piles which are going to be a strain on one's health. Healthy living and following certain principles can save one from this chronic malady.

HEARTBURN

18

One of the commonest problems faced by many people is a feeling of burning sensation in the upper part of abdomen and some people describe it as a sensation of blow torch heating his/ her insides. This is very commonly ascribed to increased acidity for which a number of factors may be operative.

But a number of people think it to be a form of indigestion. Heartburn which is present either in the upper part of abdomen or behind the breast bone has a number of causes. It is more of an uncomfortable sensation and there is not much of pain. The sufferer's hands often describe it as up and down movements over the chest. When heart burn becomes very severe, it becomes rather an uncomfortable painful experience.

A number of bizarre statements are made by the sufferers to explain their symptoms. Some may say that they feel 'as if they are on fire while others have complained of a feeling of fire coming out of their mouth.'

A large number of people all over the world suffer from it. Some degree of sensation of heartburn is felt to greater or lesser extent by most of the people. To some these symptoms are so mild that they do not require any notice, while in others they may become very distressing.

A number of factors ranging from increased intra-abdominal pressure, obesity to change in posture like bending while gardening, lifting of heavy objects, use of fried, spicy, acidic foods, excessive smoking, tea, coffee and alcohol will also give rise to sensation of heartburn.

Smoking is an important culprit. It increases acidity by raising volume of gastric secretions. Same is true of people who chew tobacco and its related products producing a number of ill effects.

In some, heartburn is accompanied by the appearance of some fluid either salty or bitter in taste in the mouth. Many complain of regurgitation of acidic sour gastric contents in the mouth.

Heartburn is normally present in great percentage of pregnant women and in some the symptoms may be very troublesome. Mostly it is experienced during the early months of pregnancy or in late months. The heartburn developing in the early months has little relation to posture and is often not affected by the use of antacids. In contrast to this the heartburn in late months is related to regurgitation of acid, meals and posture adopted by the woman. But the relieving point is that all these women get relief from heartburn after the delivery of the child.

A number of people note heartburn when lying in bed, on turning to the right side but not to the left. Invariably use of antacids gives relief to sufferers of heartburn, while conversely the use of citrus fruit juices or smoking worsens their symptoms.

But how heartburn is produced? Looking at the problem, we observe that when a person ingests some irritants such as excess of condiments, alcohol, tobacco or drugs (which are gastric irritant) there is generally inflammation not only of the stomach lining but also of the oesophagus giving rise to a form of burning sensation. This type of involvement occurs as a result of constant and regular injury to the mucosal lining of the sensitive individuals.

Similarly, when the acidity in the stomach is raised, food may regurgitate into the oesophagus giving rise to a form of oesophagitis (inflammation) and because of this the mucosa of the oesophagus becomes sensitive to even dilute acid in the stomach so that the gastric contents may produce a sensation of burning behind the breast bone. This unpleasant sensation burning in character is what is known as heart burn.

There may or may not be any regurgitation of food either into the mouth or pharynx and the degree of acidity may not always determine the presence of heart burn.

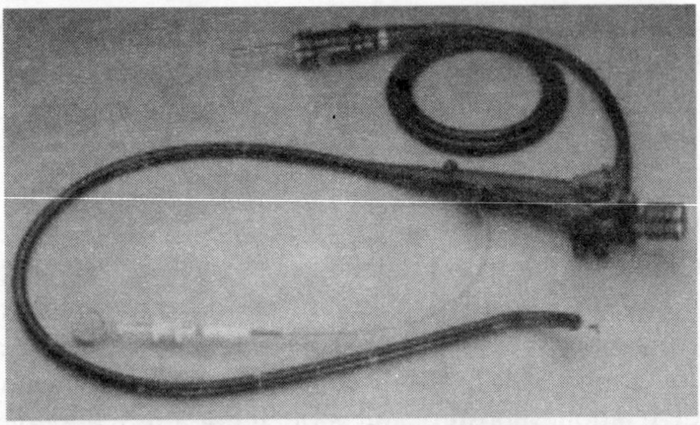

Gastroduodenofibre scope

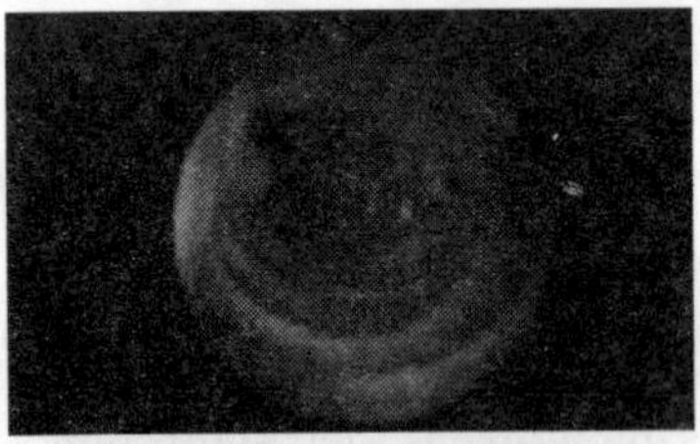

Normal Duodenum

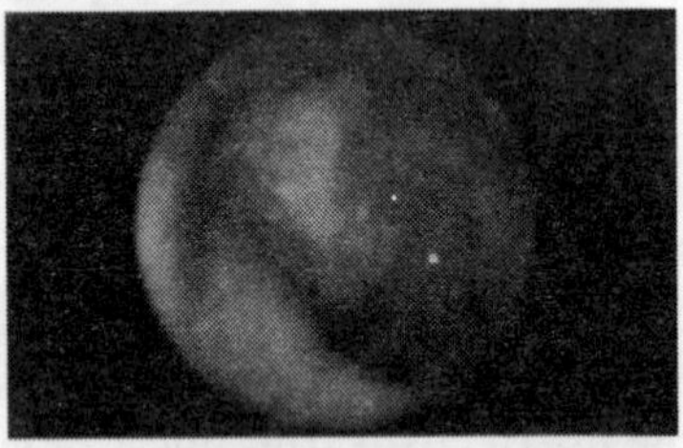

Duodenal Ulcer

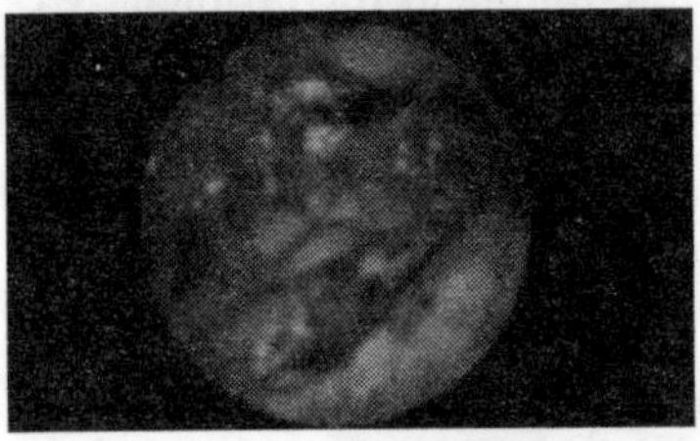

Acute Gastric Ulcer

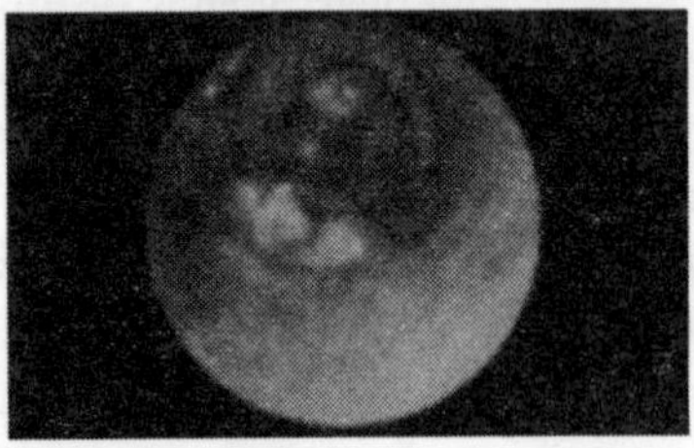

Gastric Ulcer

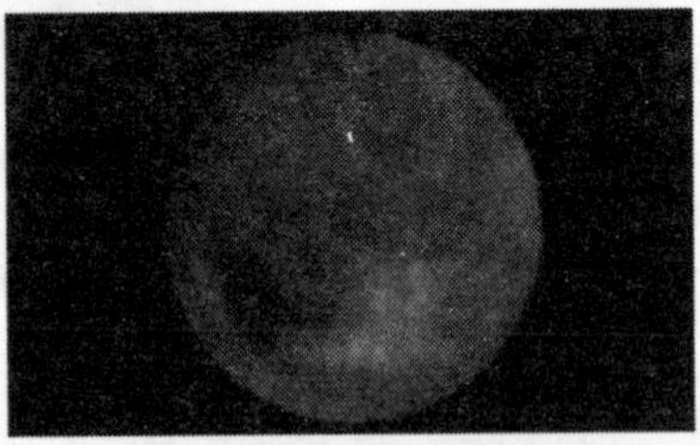

Oesophagea Cancer

Views of Stomach, Oesophagus, Duodenum in Diseases through Endoscope.

Conditions like anaemia, gastric carcinoma where acidity is low also produce a burning sensation. So the factor of increased acidity is not always there.

An important factor responsible for heartburn is the presence of reflux at the lower end of oesophagus which means the flow of gastric contents into the oesophagus and this is dependent to a large extent on the competency of the mechanism which controls the reflux. Oesophageal reflux, if it is small, may produce no symptoms but when it is substantial, oesophagitis with associated symptoms results. The normal or abnormal occurrence of reflux is dependent to a large extent on the competency of the sphincter at the lower end of oesophagus. Naturally if there is dysfunction of the sphincter, reflux will occur. This will be further accentuated by bending, lying or lifting heavy weight, factors which increase the reflux. This would be more severe in those who consume hot spicy/fatty foods and that is why some physicians label this as 'hot-fat-heart burn'.

Rise of intra-abdominal pressure due to any factor like obesity or even pregnancy shall squeeze the stomach and push the stomach contents to travel into the oesophagus resulting into a combination of either lower chest or upper abdominal pain which may come on and off with dramatic suddenness. There is not only a burning sensation but a feeling of food sitting like a lump in the chest or throat.

As material is refluxed from below, the food which enters from above may also predispose to oesophageal damage by acting in league with material from below. Thus strong tea, coffee, citrus juices and alcoholic drinks worsen the problem. Hot liquids sting their gullet and these people may perforce have to let their drinks cool before taking them.

Hiatus hernia is another condition in which heartburn is very frequent and many a lay person has often considered it synonymous with it. This is not exactly correct. Reflux may exist independent of hiatus and vice-versa, though both may coexist in many sufferers of heartburn.

Let us look as to how hiatus hernia results? Normally, the partition separating the abdomen from the thorax has several openings and the most important is the hiatus through which the food pipe or oesophagus passes to which it is loosely attached. In obese middle aged and elderly people, this attachment may weaken so that herniation of the stomach and oesophagus may occur.

Most of such people have no symptoms and may be discovered accidentally. As the sphincter at the lower end is loose, it produces free flow of acid resulting into oesophagitis. Similarly, there may be mechanical factor of stomach contents leaking back into the oesophagus or minor acidic secretions may leak from the stomach into the oesophagus so that its lining finds it difficult to tolerate. At the same time the lining of the mucosa may become so inflammed that it irritates and becomes sensitive to even ordinary foods which a person consumes.

Out of these the mechanical factor is difficult to control. There is generally incompetency of the mechanism controlling reflux as well as tone of the sphincter at the lower end with the result that whenever there is any factor which raises intra-abdominal pressure like wearing of tight clothes, belts, garters, obesity, etc. or the person either lies down or bends over especially after a heavy meal or even breathes deeply or even sighs, etc. there is regurgitation of abdominal contents into oesophagus.

All such people have heart burnafter meals especially after seasonal and heavy food and those who wear tight clothes they complain of discomfort while bending during course of home work, or lifting heavy weight or straining. When these people lie down after food at night there may be discomfort which wakens up the patient and he or she may have to sit up. Often it becomes essential to differentiate whether the symptoms in any particular person are due to reflux or hiatus. Since very distressing symptoms may be present, yet there may be no hiatus whatsoever and it is basically reflux from an incompetent sphincter which requires attention.

The diagnosis of hiatus hernia is made by taking Barium X-rays after keeping the patient in certain positions. These pictures determine the capacity of the individual to herniate and define whether herniation is continuous or intermittent.

Commonly the prone horizontal or head-down position or antigravity position with head tilted 10° down is employed. To show the presence or absence of reflux the person may be required either to straight raise the leg or touch the toes or squat from the standing position. Reflux of food, etc. is demonstrated in one of these positions or may be the position in which the patient gets his symptoms. Another method is to measure the pressure at the lower end of oesophagus as well as in stomach. Subsequently oesophagoscopy may be required.

Surprisingly women are more liable to suffer from heartburn as compared to men. As long as heartburn is mild it does not cause much concern. But it is really the people who get symptoms frequently or where these are distressing that it causes concern. In the beginning these people used to get relief by the use of antacids but now they do not get it. Their symptoms get worse when they lie in bed at night. Use of tight clothes, garters and belts especially in women worsen their symptoms and similarly when they try to bend forward or lift something heavy from floor they feel quite uncomfortable.

In contrast to the factor of hiatus hernia, one must not ignore a very common ailment which is equally responsible for heartburn. This common ailment is peptic ulcer which comprises of either a gastric or duodenal ulcer. The most common complaint of these patients is pain or burning sensation localised to the upper part of abdomen in the central region. Pain occurs when the stomach is empty. The sufferer complains of pain which may be in the form of uneasiness or a gnawing sensation. It is related to food. While a case of gastric ulcer gets pain after taking food (food-pain-relief) a case of duodenal ulcer gets relief after taking food (Food-Relief-Pain). Such people have a history of getting up at night because of pain. Oesophagitis, a form of inflammation of the food pipe may be acute or chronic. There is discomfort or pain in the lower part of breast bone when a person eats solid food, takes hot drinks or strong alcohol. There is often an ulcer which is associated with a hiatus hernea.

A case of cancer of the oesophagus (Food pipe) may complain of difficulty or discomfort on swallowing and pain occurs rather late. Regurgitation of food also occurs sooner or later. Some patients may only complain of something odd sticking in the pit of stomach.

Worm infestation is a very common problem all over the world. People who suffer from various worm infestations (round worm, hook worm, tape worm), often have a feeling of something eating them inside the abdomen, a form of discomfort, nausea and vomiting.

So one would appreciate that a sufferer from heartburn may have a number of ailments ranging from hiatus hernia, oesophagitis, peptic ulcer to worm infestation. Every person who comes with these various complaints must be subjected to stools examination, serological tests, barium studies of oesophagus, stomach and duodenum. An endoscopy is a must and from suspicious places, biopsy be taken.

Once the diagnosis has been arived, appropriate treatment must be instituted under the advice of physician.

The next question is as to how to manage sufferers from heartburn where no organic disease is present.

In large majority of such people, provided proper precautions are taken it is not difficult to be free from the symptoms of fire inside. One thing is clear that heartburn seems to result from combination of a number of factors. The mucous lining of the oesophagus (gullet) may be hypersensitive and secondly the irritant may be vicious. So one has to look for all these factors.

Basically reflux is influenced by gravity since in the case stomach is at higher level than the oesophagus, the heartburn will be perpetuated. So the sufferer must avoid too frequent bending or stooping. If these people have to pick something from the floor or even tie their shoe laces, instead of stooping they should preferably be sitting on their knees and not bending forward.

The housewife must use long handled brush or broom for sweeping or dusting the house. Similarly, long handled tools be employed for gardening.

Avoid the use of low chair after meals, since this will tend to bring the symptoms of heartburn.

Do not lie flat in bed after meals. Raise the head end of the bed or lower the foot end. A pile of pillows or blankets may be used to produce the right angle for the back. Similarly, these people when going on a journey should preferably use a small pillow behind their back on their seats.

It is preferable to use a special type of bed which raises the head end of bed to specific angles. Some people find using a 6 inches block under the head end of the bed to be very useful. Similarly, it may be desirable to raise the upper half of the mattress or pillows. Another useful method in addition to sleeping propped up, is to employ a wedged pillow at the head of the bed and another beneath the knees.

Since reflux may be due to chemical irritation, it is very important to change the food habits of the person. All fried, hot spicy food, be avoided. Use of strong tea, coffee or alcohol be restricted and only weak beverages taken. Let the stomach be not full. Take small feeds but at more frequent intervals. Avoid taking of food 2-3 hours before going to bed.

Rich, heavy meals must be avoided as heavy, rich, fatty food is likely to reflux during the night. Let dinner be a simple affair. In the words of a leading physician, 'smaller-less fatty and sweet meals are recommended for such people'.

Avoid strong acidic drinks. Coffee and smoking should preferably be cut down.

Pressure over the stomach worsens the symptoms in a sufferer of heartburn. The symptoms of heartburn which occur during pregnancy usually improve after the delivery when the abdominal pressure has fallen.

Similarly, the use of tight clothes, corsets and belts should be avoided. Those women who get heartburn must see that their clothing is loose and no undue pressure is applied over the abdomen.

Overweight must be curbed. Reduction in weight relieves the pressure over the stomach by reducing intra-abdominal pressure and ensures relief to a large extent.

And if general measures detailed above do not help, then small meals accompanied by the use of antacids often help. Take antacids before heartburn begins and do not wait for it to begin, since when it starts it means that the oesophagus has already been irritated and inflammed and the whole vicious process is being perpetuated.

But one point is quite clear and that is antacids help when taken before and after meals which should be small. One must ensure rest to the inflammed oesophagus by reducing the amount of stomach contents which may reflux. Majority of sufferers from heartburn respond quickly to the use of antacids. Quick acting antacids are really very useful. It is better to take liquid form of antacids rather than tablets, since they shall give relief earlier.

And lastly an important aspect of this malady is the state of fear and stress due to the distressing heartburn. What an individual requires is reassurance as to howsoever unpleasant the symptoms may be, they shall not prove dangerous.

General measures especially as regard to food, weight, strong drinks, postures adopted while sleeping and use of antacids, all help such people. Most such people do well and can go on leading a normal life. It is an occasional case of heartburn with hiatus hernia who fails to improve with the general measures and surgical help is required which gives relief in majority of people.

To conclude heartburn is a distressing symptom complex dependent on the oesophageal reflux as well as number of other factors but it is one condition which should not alarm the sufferer, since properly managed, relief is obtained quickly.

19 EMOTIONS AND GASTROINTESTINAL TRACT

Emotions play great role in the proper functioning of a person's gastrointestinal tract. Anybody with a functional disorder always has a psychological conflict at the root of his/her problems and these conflicts may be at either conscious or subconscious level and the person may not be aware of it.

Conflicts of varying nature and emotional unheavals go a long way in effecting a change in person's attitude towards his/her bodily functions. Of all the bodily functions gastrointestinal tract may be the one which is effected to a large extent by all the individuals inner conflicts and various emotions ranging from anxiety, nervousness to depression.

Emotional disturbances may produce loss of appetite, vomiting, dyspepsia, heartburn or even looseness of bowels. Nervousness produces haste in the stomach so that the alimentary tract tries to hasten the food. Over sensitiveness in a person results in a sensitive stomach. There are alterations in the acid secretions, mucus, lysozyme and friability of the stomach mucosa, all due to emotional disturbances. At the same time both the small and large bowels also react in an abnormal manner to the various emotions.

Anxiety is normal reaction of the body to a state of stress and shall be evident in all types of people normally to a small or large extent, depending on the individual's threshold and reactions. Most of the people tolerate anxiety but there are a number of such people who perpetually remain over-anxious, high strung and tense. Gastrointestinal response in such people is very variable. There is usually a feeling of dryness of the mouth, loss of appetite, nausea, vomiting, belching bringing out lot of air and often a diarrhoea which is watery and too frequent.

Some of these symptoms are quite evident when a person is going for an important engagement, before an interview or an examination. Symptoms of anxiety and gastrointestinal response are generally a reaction but to a large extent are over reaction to an emotion which is normally present. Mild symptoms tend to disappear as the stressful situation is over. But even sometimes the altered functions of an ailment might be brought into prominence because of the emotional upheaval.

Similarly, frustration shall give rise to a voracious appetite, since lot of such people derive pleasure from large quantities of food. Conversely, a dissatisfied mind shall always find the food to be unpleasant. When a person is depressed it is his/her entire mood which is changed. There is overall slackness of activity both physical and mental and even faculties of thinking are affected. In other words the person not only feels ill but also looks ill. Zest and drive, all are lost. The individual looses appetite and develops a distaste towards food. In addition, there is lack of sleep and the person not only finds it difficult to go to sleep at night but also gets up in the early hours of the morning. Sometimes, the person complains of indigestion, abdominal distension, gaseousness, constipation and even abdominal pain.

Most of the sufferers from abdominal complaints are really victims of hypochondriasis. They are always plagued by imaginary disorders of gastointestinal tract. This sort of abdominal neuroses is the bane of all sort of people but more of intelligent people, since once they get it they manifest in a more striking manner. Compared to this group, the unlettered and poorer people may have less and more vague symptoms.

The neurotic response of these sufferers is more of a compensatory reaction to the worries, disappointments, frustrations and boredoms, etc. Basically, such people have a neurotic personality and of rather sensitive nature and suffer from obsessional traits. Their symptoms range from dyspepsia, flatulence, abdominal distension and vague abdominal pains. Akin to a neurotic personality, a hysterical person generally a young woman, may present with odd gastrointestinal symptoms. There may be persistent vomiting, vague indigestion and abdominal distension. Loss of appetite is present in a great number of such people.

Some of the hysterics may complain of pain in the abdomen which is generally constant and is unaccompanied by any emotions or feelings over his/her face. Pain is never constant and wanders from one part of the abdomen to another.

In fact it is really a problem to manage such people. It has been rightly said that gastrointestinal disturbances in no way reflect a disturbance in a single portion of the gastrointestinal tract but are due to wide spread alterations in the functions of the digestive tract.

Thus anything starting from disagreeable taste, functional regurgitation, vomiting, belching, aerophagy, emotional diarrhoea, irritable colon to peptic ulcer, ulcerative colitis may result from situations of stress and emotional unheavals or may be just functional in origin. The number of such people is on the increase and they are making rounds of doctor's clinics with some of these disorders where emotions are playing havoc with their system. Let us look at some of these problems in a little more detail.

Loss of Appetite

It is a very common condition, in fact the commonest which is associated with emotional stress or trauma. Periods of depression, failure in the examination or a love affair not proceeding to a satisfactory course, absence of congenial atmosphere either at home or in office, financial difficulties or any emotional tension leads to nothing but lack of desire for food. One often comes across people not taking food even for days together just because they do not feel like taking it. Uneasiness in the upper abdomen and lack of interest in food with resultant loss of appetite occurs in a great majority of students with pre-examination tension and disappears after the successful completion of the test.

As long as a person has only temporary loss of appetite it may not cause much anxiety but when it goes further characterised by not only loss of appetite and loss of weight with subsequent emaciation it assumes the name of condition called 'Anorexia Nervosa'. It commonly affects young adults of both the sexes but more so young women who have got a knack of refusing food and are often a cause of concern in the family. The disorder generally develops in young women who voluntarily refuse to take food due to fear of getting fat. Radical restriction of food results in wasting and emaciation.

In this condition, the patient achieves his/her aim by severely restricting coloric intake. In contrast to anorexia nervosa, there is a condition called Bulimia where patient takes large amounts of food and then brings it out by vomiting. Very often both anorexia nervosa and bulimia are considered two facets of a process aimed at losing weight. To start with, an anorexic patient refuses to eat with subsequent reduction in food intake and finally all desire for food is lost. The person may have to be coaxed to eat but this gives rise to a sense of repulsion towards food. Gradually, the person starts losing weight which generally is more than 25 per cent of the original body weight. But despite this the patient is alert and may follow exercise programmes to further reduce weight.

Due to lack of food intake, there is constipation and often use of laxatives is employed. Patient, a young woman has a distorted sense of food intake and weight control. Amenorrhoea is often present. Psychogenic factors also play a role. They are usually model children who had been well cared for. They have lacked self-confidence and been brought up under strict discipline.

As symptoms progress, the person who was previously in prime of health is now lethargic, fatigued and wasted. There is slowing of heart rate, fall of blood pressure and fall of body temperature. There is growth of downy body hair. Parotid glands become prominent. Oedema/swelling appears on the legs and feet.

Because of severe emaciation patient lies in bed listless without taking any interest in his/her self and the surrounding. Psychogenic factors also come to play their role.

Diagnosis of anorexia nervosa is based on the following criteria:

(i) Young girl generally in her twenties

(ii) Anorexia

(iii) Loss of weight

(iv) Absence of any organic disease or psychiatric illness which might account for the disease.

(v) Severe restriction of food intake whether or not accompanied by vomiting.

In addition, the person shows a picture of wasted person, lethargic and is often bed-ridden. Pulse is slow. There is fall of blood pressure. Body fat disappears and the bones protrude. Skin is dry, scaly and often yellow. Sometimes, despite the advanced stage of disease, some patients may show overactivity. Laboratory investigations show anaemia and electrolyte imbalance. Blood glucose levels fall and blood urea levels go up because of impairment of renal concentrating ability. Radiologically there is no abnormality.

Management of sufferers of anorexia nervosa requires lot of tact and patience. It is very essential to remove such a person from his/her surroundings. Gradual encouragement to take food is instituted step by step so that the person starts taking soft nutritious food. There may be slight discomfort complained of in the beginning and the person may resist attempts at feeding yet with proper persuasion, the initial resistance on the part of the person breaks. To start with, the person may require supervision at the time of feeding but once the vicious circle breaks, there is no subsequent problem. Attempt should be made to regain lost weight. Food is soft, nutritious and easily digestible. Sometimes feeding may induce abdominal discomfort.

When patient is very ill and resists attempts at feeding hospitalization may be necessary. It is equally important that oversolicitous and overanxious family members of the persons, household are kept away from him/her, so that they let the person face the realities of life boldly and with courage.

Where there is complete lack of appetite, treatment with insulin before principal meals helps in improving appetite and gaining weight. In some cases parenteral nutrition might have to be instituted.

Where psychological factors are operative, antidepressants and tranquilizers are given. But at the same time a patient of anorexia nervosa requires reassurance about the safety of eating and regaining his/her health. Prognosis in a case of anorexia nervosa is generally good. Where patient starts accepting food early gain in weight occurs while those who resist treatment complications like cardiac irregularities, intercurrent illnesses develop. Starvation accounts for death in 6 per cent of the patients. In some, psychiatric disturbances may induce suicidal tendencies. If managed properly, the patient of anorexia nervosa regains his/her health in a span of six months to one year.

Functional Vomiting

Vomiting is one complaint which always causes lot of anxiety not only in the sufferer's mind but also amongst his/her near and dear ones.

Though a number of diseases of central nervous system starting from encephalitis, meningitis and brain tumours to migraine, etc. give rise to vomiting but there are some people who suffer from it because of emotional factors. In such people the regurgitation of food occurs without any accompanying nausea or retching. The stomach is never completely emptied.

In neurotic people the emotions of fear, anxiety and digust may induce vomiting and it may be due to subconscious revival of the memory of events which are rather of an unpleasant nature.

Vomiting may be hysterical in nature which has been aptly called a form of physical defence against some intolerable situation. The sufferer generally is a young female who is in conflict with either her husband or in-laws. Similarly, there may be disturbed situations which bring out the hidden dormant emotions to the forefront and an exacerbation of the person's symptoms.

Hysterics always vomit immediately after meals in the presence of company.

The vomiting in hysterics is always accompanied by much noise. The stomach is emptied only half with the result that though such people suffer from vomiting for a number of years, their nutrition is well maintained and they do not suffer from either malnutrition or wasting.

Majority of people with functional vomiting require deft handling. Since a number of the sufferers are young women they are most of the time emotionally upset. Some may have problems with their in-laws and especially so in a joint family system, the young lady might not be getting the same sympathy and attention from her husband which she might be wishing for. In some, there is problem of sexual adjustments. Result is that vomiting occurs and the young woman becomes the centre of attention of the whole family. No diet is known to influence vomiting. It may follow a full meal or may be only after a glass of milk. In both cases, the vomiting is quite frequent.

The patient produces loud barborygmi and noises which are heard across the room. Management of hysterical vomiting is difficult and requires careful handling going into details of personal and family history.

Water Brash

It is another common symptom in which at a certain interval after a meal, varying in different people and constant in some, an uncomfortable feeling of constriction is felt behind the breast bone. There is accompanying excessive salivation. Soon these people being out mouthfuls of clear fluid just like water containing some mucus and are almost compelled to pour this fluid out.

This degree of excessive salivation which is very profuse, comes from the upper part, is just watery and contains no food at all. Neurotic persons suffer more from water brash. It is interesting to observe these people bringing out lot of saliva without much efforts and that too by the mouthfuls. Some may complain of a brassy or a peculiar taste in their mouth. Except for the aesthetic undesirability such people have no other problem and even require no treatment.

Nervous Dyspepsia

It is said that if there was a window on the stomach by which it can be examined at will then probably one shall be able to see the various emotional ups and downs of the individual being reflected there. In short, the mucosa and secretions of the stomach can act as emotional barometer of the person's stress and strain.

Stress effects organs in a physiologic manner by producing ischemia, decreased or excessive secretions or movements. In fact frustration, anger, happiness and all sorts of conflicts shall evoke a different response in the stomach. Anger, resentment and hostility not only increase the gastric secretions, do rapid emptying but also make mucosa of the stomach look angry or friable.

All these emotional outbursts with their resultant effects are closely related to individual's digestion and indigestion. Emotions like anxiety, anger frustration, depression, guilt sensations, overwork and fatigue, all give rise to indigestion. Similarly, such people have abdominal discomfort, waxing and waning during the day without any specific relation on the type of food eaten. This discomfort has a direct bearing to either anxiety, worry, depression or even any undesirable excitement. These are the people who are accustomed to swallowing lot of air, belching, making noises and even suffer from not only a sense of fullness but also gaseous distension of abdomen. Sufferers from excessive gas formation have what is called a 'gaseous personality' and have multiplicity of symptoms varying from anxiety to palpitation.

The symptoms of nervous dyspepsia go well with an emotionally labile personality. The symptoms referred to other systems are bizarre. There may be complaints of headache and lack of sleep. The person may appear to be of worrying type paying attention to his/her body the whole day and worrying about a few minor ailments all the time.

Many such people go with imaginary complaints from one doctor to another doctor, trying all types of home remedies, the advertised drugs and shall not be satisfied with any single treatment. In fact such people develop a form of fixation complex as far as their stomach or digestion is concerned.

No doubt, such person requires thorough investigations which generally show no abnormality. Since most of such people are always exaggerating their complaints they require to be reassured and managed sympathetically. With proper advice, guidance and psychological work-up, it is not difficult to manage such people.

Along with nervous dyspepsia some degree of spasm at the lower end of food pipe may be present (cardiospasm). A feeling of something sticking and a little burning sensation may be complained of. Such people are generally considered to be rather dry in nature, humorless, suspicious, non-committal and defensive rather than aggressive in their dealings with people in day to day problems. Moreover, these are the people who try to suppress rather than express their conflicts and feelings. In a nutshell they ruminate, brood and this is shown not only by their oesophageal dysfunction but also by dyspepsia. It has been righly remarked that unhappiness, commotion, overexcitement are the greatest cause of nervous indigestion.

Before any conclusions are arrived at, the patient must be thoroughly investigated and any organic ailment excluded.

Once the patient has been declared to be having no abnormality he should be reassured. Symptomatic relief be given by use of antacids and a little sedative. Psychiatric help can be sought and treatment advised accordingly.

Emotions, Stress and Peptic Ulcer

As said earlier, stomach is one organ which acts as a barometer of an individual's emotional upheavals. Tensions of varying type take their toll on this organ. Stress of modern day civilization is responsible to large extent in producing picture of an ulcer in the stomach. Though number of other factors shall play their role but stress is an important factor.

Shakespeare in his play "Julius Caesar" has very well illustrated this aspect. He has rightly said (Act I, Scene 8), "You Cassius hath a lean and hungry look: he thinks too much" and in these words Shakespeare was probably defining the modern day 'Cassisus'—one who is always worked-up about something; frets and grumbles about everything whether it is his job, family or even the society in general. This is one man who always finds some fault or the other in everything and always tries to achieve perfection. This modern day character is the prototype of Shakespear's Cassius and one who is more prone to get ulcers. But this is the personality of an ulcer prone individual, a person of slender and thin built with a built up which is characterized by rigidity, over consciousness and even intolerance. People with ulcer are the ones who seem to reflect disturbances in their inner self than in the outside world.

The effects of stress are variable. Stress concerned with one's place of work, nature and type of work along with the living conditions also have a bearing on the problem of ulcer. Men in the Army and Navy who have to be away from their homes for very long periods at a stretch are always more prone to get ulcers.

In a study amongst the men of Royal Navy it was found that the incidence of ulcer amongst the ratings was very high, since these people were exposed to climatic extremes of heat and cold, to extremes of heat and humidity in situations such as the engine and boiler room; the increased degree of responsibility, long periods of separation from their families coupled with anxiety about their homes and family problems. Broken homes and domestic unhappiness, the financial anxieties, the pressure of group behaviour, allure of foreign ports, technical hazards and environmental tensions, the mental demands of new technology and physical demands of a tight routine all went a long way in increasing the problem of ulcer amongst these people.

So, in a way emotions put a great demand on the stomach of a person. But all said and done, it would be difficult to say whether there is really an ulcer personality except that these people are abnormally anxious, aggressive and have excessive obsessional trends and are more prone to anxiety, dependence, guilt feeling and are easily frightened by slightly difficult situations.

Pain in Abdomen

Pain in abdomen is one of the most disturbing complaints which always requires attention. Most of the sufferers from this malady are having chronic abdominal pain and relief is what the sufferer desires. Pain in abdomen may be due to various causes related to the organs present in the abdomen or it may be a referred pain due to either diseases of the heart, lung or nervous system.

Every pain in abdomen requires thorough investigations from the point of view of excluding organic ailments including parasites, ulcer, small or large bowel disorders, liver and gall bladder ailments. But despite the serious nature of the cause of pain in abdomen, there is still a number of people where the pain in abdomen is functional. The commonest cause of such pain is due to anxiety, nervous tension or even hysteria. When it is of functional origin there are also disturbances of bodily function like fatigue, loss of energy, zest as well as a feeling of exhaustion and weakness. Such persons have flatulence, dyspepsia, loss of taste for food, consciousness of bowel functions and altered bowel habits. Many such individuals suffer from a feeling of guilt, a sense of helplessness and worthlessness. Often the abdominal discomfort has been associated with unpleasant events in life like retirement, loss of power, position and prestige.

Pain due to functional causes is vague, present either in the whole of abdomen or often just to the left midline in the upper abdomen.

To start with, the pain in such people is vague, mild but gradually when it becomes established, the person starts taking unusual interest in his/her bodily functions worrying all the time about either his/her dirty tongue or some imaginary abdominal complaints. Rightly it has been commented that the individual's emotional shock is being reflected in his/her abdomen.

All persons coming with pain abdomen require thorough investigations and only after excluding the organic causes, the diagnosis of functional abdominal pain associated with emotional stress (at a conscious or subconscious level) is made.

Functional Disorders related to Organic Diseases of the Abdomen

Not only there is a correlation between bodily disease and emotional factors but there are a number of organic abdominal diseases like duodenal ulcer and inflammatory bowel disturbances which bear a close relationship to emotional stress or strain.

Stress is one factor which has been blamed to play great part in the causation of ulcers. A number of experimental studies have tended to show that stress ulcers are observed in laboratory rats subjected to number of various stimuli and similarly they have been observed in animals who have been immobilized in close fitting cages, thus inducing a feeling of rage and helplessness.

In humans a higher incidence of occupational, emotional and financial crises has been observed in sufferers of chronic duodenal ulcer. Feelings of anxiety, pent up anger and hostility are much more common in ulcer sufferers who are also hypersecretors of acid.

Not only the stomach but the small and large bowels also react to stress in different ways. Irritable colon occurs in regular fashion coinciding with periods of stress and emotional strain.

One rough estimate puts that almost every human being occasionally experiences colonic dysfunction at sometime or other in his life as a result of physical or emotional stress. A significantly greater incidence of stressful situations is present in sufferers of irritable bowel.

During periods of emotional conflict changes in motility, mucus secretions and vascularity of the gut have been found in sufferers from this malady. In fact a close relationship between bowel functions and emotions has been postulated and readily accepted. Bowels participate in the overall body response to the emotions. In addition to bowel dysfunction, there may be flushing, excessive sweating, fatigue and lack of sleep.

Though no specific characteristics can be ascribed to such people but a great majority of the sufferers are rigid, aggressive, compulsive and cold in their relationship with others. They are midway between normal and psychoneurotic personality. Sufferers from irritable bowel get their symptoms aggravated during periods of hostile behaviour and it is possible that these people are exhibiting their aggressive feelings through their bowels.

Similarly, sufferers from inflammatory bowel disorders like ulcerative colitis have been known to have psychogenic factors operative and worsening of their symptoms during an emotional upheaval.

The typical personality of such a person is that of a sensitive individual, timid in nature who is unable to act to aggressive situations. Such people both men and women may view their mothers as powerful and overwhelming figures who set high standards and made them feel helpless and dependent on either their mother or one of the parents. A disturbance in this relationship may bring on an exacerbation in their symptoms.

Basically such people are cold and do not develop warm relationship with others. Another hypothesis is that ulcerative colitis occurs in persons with immature and defective egos. But the symptoms in all such organic ailments are aggravated by stressful situations and both the organic and functional symptoms overlap so much that there is often a problem in differentiating between the two forms of ailment.

It is only brings home the importance of psychological factors whether primary or secondary which either initiate or complicate an abdominal dysfunction.

Management

The management of people with emotional disorders accompanying or causing gastrointestinal symptoms require a sympathetic understanding of the person and his/her psyche. It also cannot be denied that some of the disorders of the digestive system may just be shown by symptoms other than related to gastrointestinal tract. Recognition of the functional aspect of the disorder is very important. There may be certain positive features suggesting a functional disturbance in the form of functional vomiting, aerophagia, excessive belching, etc. The person's complaints are rather inconstant, vague and may be waxing and waning in bizarre fashion over a period of years. The emotional liability is more predominant in the individual's actions and behaviour. There may be complaints ascribed to other systems like increase in pulse and heart rate, excessive sweating and flushing, etc. There are often features of excessive tiredness, headache, insomnia, numbness in the hands, and feet, tremors, etc. In fact the person either shows undue concern about his/her ailment or is unduly worried about a symptom or complaint which is rather of very minor nature.

Many people are hesitant to disclose their correct emotional history as well as background. Circumstantial evidence has to be obtained from their socio-economic background, educational and cultural influences and the nature of stress as well as strain. Degrees of anxiety, depression, emotional conflicts either at home or place of work be looked into. A broken home, unhappy sex life, failure in love relationship, tensions at place of work, etc., all may be contributing to the various adverse life situations.

But the evidence in favour of a functional disorder producing gastrointestinal symptoms is generally circumstantial. The final conclusions are arrived at by examination and excluding evidence in favour of organic diseases which could produce these symptoms.

Detailed laboratory investigations including X-rays of the ailmentary tract, utrasound of abdomen must be done before a diagnosis of a functional disorder of the gastrointestinal tract is made. One must stress here the point that labelling an organic disease as a functional one can be very dangerous so a correct assessment of such people is very important. It is a long and laborious process, since the road to recovery is slow but the ultimate success is always there provided patience, sympathy and understanding of an individual's problem is undertaken.

In fact a sort of relationship is cultivated which ensures confidence on the part of the sufferer.

All such persons require thorough understanding of their problem coupled by reassurance. Most of them are either anxious or depressed. The person is encouraged to express his/her pent up feelings in a way that he/she unburdens the mind of troubles which might be weighing heavily upon his/her mind. Conflicts at place of work or in the family must be tackled and solved to the mutual satisfaction of all. The person has to be impressed that a certain amount of tension or stress is a normal part of every day life and one has to put up with it. Hope about getting relief from the person's undesirable situations must be kindled.

Rest, exercise and outdoor activities must be cultivated so that the person's mind is taken away from his/her imaginary problems. Auto-suggestion, auto-relaxation, hypnosis and meditation techniques are quite helpful. Good nourishing food must be enjoined upon to be taken in adequate quantities. In addition to psychotherapy, diet and general measures, drugs in the form of sedatives and pain relieving ones are employed. But this is best left in the hands of treating physician.

Successful management of all the persons with functional disorders depends to a large extent on taking persons away from the emotional tensions or conflicts and understanding of the problems which cannot be changed. Long and needless worry about minor complaints must be ignored.

Person must learn to live with his upheavals and conflicts in life. A judicious and calm attitude shall go along way in helping a person to come out of his/her problems.

PAINFUL SWALLOWING 20

Swallowing is a normal physiological process and is governed by a number of factors. A number of people suffer from either painful swallowing or difficulty in swallowing which is often a cause of anxiety.

Oesophagus (food pipe) connects the oropharynx to the stomach. It itself is composed of smooth muscle and it is the coordinated action of muscular layers of the body of the food pipe which helps in the passage of the food boluses and liquids from the upper end to the stomach. A series of reflexes constitute the normal act of swallowing which is a painless process. The normal process of swallowing may be interfered with either due to functional or pathological conditions. There may be difficulty in swallowing because of the pain during the act. Painful swallowing is a condition which cannot be ignored and a number of conditions may be responsible for it.

Associated with painful swallowing is a condition also called difficulty in swallowing, i.e., dysphagia which is a Greek word. From the lay person's point of view both painful swallowing and difficulty in swallowing are almost synonymous to each other since the conditions responsible for one intermingle with those of other.

The common condition in the oropharyngeal area include painful conditions of the tongue, oral cavity, acute tonsillitis, acute laryngitis and neuromuscular disorders. It is not difficult to assess the inflammatory conditions, since these are acute, person suffers from toxaemia and fever. But very often neuromuscular disorders may produce difficulty in swallowing, nasal regurgitation of liquids, gagging or coughing due to accumulation of food in the pharynx and its spillage into the trachea. This type of picture results in those suffering from neurological disorders like motor neurone disease or viral encephalitis which is an acute condition.

Painful swallowing is due to various causes ranging from infections, trauma following instrumentation, foreign body getting lodged in the food pipe, diverticular (small pouches) to malignancy.

Trauma is an important cause and is most often due to procedure like endoscopy. Here the problem is temporary and lasts only for a few days. It has also been seen in patients of asthma who have perforce swallowed small live fish and these people have a feeling of rawness in throat and difficulty in swallowing.

Mild degree of inflammation of the food pipe is often seen in those who suffer from severe degree of respiratory tract infections. In fact a number of serious ailments like tuberculosis, sepsis, syphilis and inflammatory conditions of larynx, throat may present with pain while swallowing. Patients of diabetes and those who are on broad spectrum antibiotics and immunosuppressive drugs where Candida and a number of viruses may invade the body, these people show white patches of monilial infection in their food pipe. These are the ones who complain of difficulty in swallowing. A careful assessment of patients of AIDS and those suffering from cancer in the body will show that these people who are often debilitated, undernourished and wasted, show almost the same picture, since their body resistance is low and they fall easy prey to various infections.

A foreign body may be an important cause and produces severe degree of pain during the act of swallowing. All types of foreign bodies are known to be impacted in the upper part of food pipe especially in young children but a fish bone swallowed during a meal is a common cause in adults and it should be specially kept in mind when eating fish and proper care taken.

Young females who suffer from severe anaemia especially iron deficiency along with glossitis may complain of food sticking in the throat and pain during the act of swallowing. This often

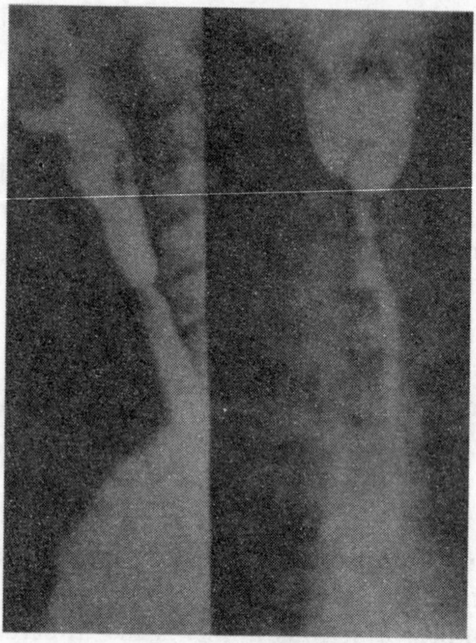

Web in a case of anaemia with difficulty in swallowing

causes a panic reaction in such people. It should be looked into. A barium study of food pipe along with endoscopy shall show the presence of a web in the upper part of food pipe. These webs disappear once anaemia is adequately treated.

Gastro-oesophageal reflux where the contents of stomach spill into the food pipe may produce not only heartburn but also substernal discomfort as well as difficulty in swallowing. People suffering from arthritis who are on anti-inflammatory drugs like Brufen, Voveran, Indomethacin, etc. and steroids are likely to suffer from ulceration in food pipe. Prolonged and severe reflux may lead to stricture formation, resulting in not only painful swallowing but also difficulty in swallowing.

Oesophageal spasm in young women may be an early sign of hysteria. A number of diseases unrelated to gastrointestinal tract such as myasthenia gravis, motor neurone disease, connective tissue disorders are known to produce severe degree of spasm as well as pain during the act of swallowing.

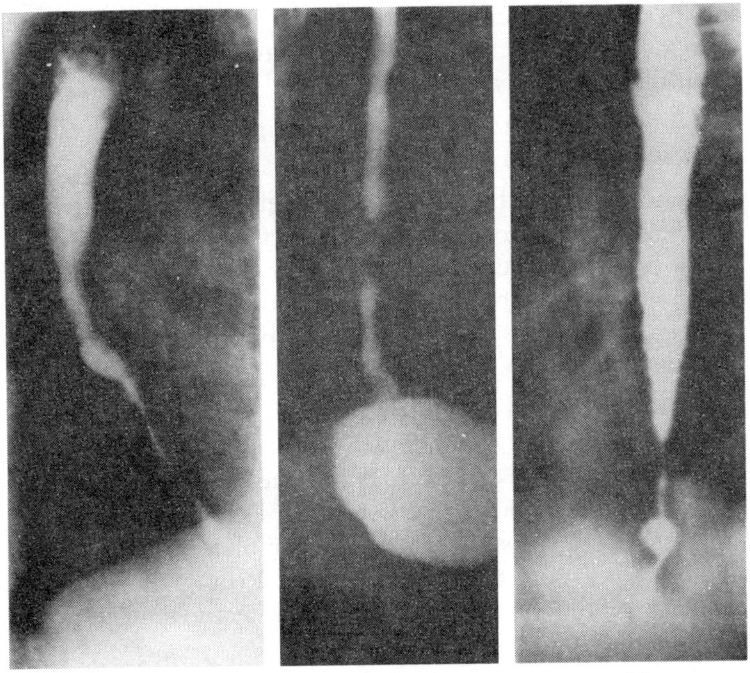

(a) (b) (c)

Painfull Swallowing/Dysphagia

Barium study of food pipe showing (a) Carcinoma involving middle and lower third, (b) Middle of food pipe, (c) Lower end of food pipe. Notice narrowing of that part

As said earlier, painful swallowing and difficulty in swallowing almost intermingle and the same causes may be operative in both.

People who come complaining of difficulty in swallowing especially in upper part, in them precancerous and cancerous conditions should be seriously considered. It is more so in a person after the age of 50. Difficulty in swallowing solids is the patient's first complaint which may or may not be painful. To start with, this difficulty is encountered only for a short period but progresses gradually over a period of weeks. Now there is pain either in the breast bone, back or in the neck. Swallowing is invariably painful. This is especially so on swallowing hot liquids and is often ignored. Progressive weight loss with regurgitation of food which is often bloodstained should alarm the person about the seriousness of the condition.

So if any person suffers from either painful or difficulty in swallowing it should not be ignored.

When the problem comes acutely, it often favours neurological disorder (Bulbar Polio, Infective Polyneuritis) while a slow progressive course favours cancer. When the problem is only transient and of short duration an inflammatory process is thought of but if the problem goes on from weeks to months it must be viewed with suspicion.

The type of food causing obstruction also helps in making a diagnosis. Difficulty in swallowing only solid foods occurs in mechanical causes like cancer. But as the condition progresses obstruction to liquids as well results. The whole process is progressive and the sufferer not only complains of pain at that site but also to something sticking there. Regurgitation of food contents and blood in them shall be other features suggestive of carcinoma of food pipe.

A word here about two neurological disorders. Myasthenia gravis is one condition where patient gets difficulty in swallowing and this increases as the day passes but sometimes there is spontaneous improvement especially when rest has been given to muscles of deglutation. In contrast to this, cases of motor neurone disease, the difficulty in swallowing is slowly progressive and there is no change in its course.

Above is a brief description of some of the important causes responsible for painful swallowing/difficulty in swallowing.

Any person who has the problem must consult his/her doctor so that treatment can be instituted at the earliest.

Every case of such nature must be subjected to radiological study of food pipe. It may show a stricture/web/narrowing of food pipe.

Oesophagoscopy is another procedure where the food pipe is visualised and diagnosis arrived at. This procedure is often combined with biopsy from the site of lesion.

Treatment and management of any such case is best left in the hands of a competent physician. Dysphagia/painful swallowing is a symptom complex of both local as well as general diseases. Treatment has to be planned, depending on the various causes. If you get either a painful swallowing or difficulty in swallowing, do not ignore it. It may be harbinger of a serious ailment.

21 COMMON GASTROINTESTINAL PROBLEMS

Besides the problems of gas formation, constipation, loose bowels, heart burn and emotional upheavals, etc., there are still some common problems which deserve attention from a lay person's point of view. Let us look at some of them.

Stomatitis

It means inflammation of the mouth and is caused by bacterial viral and fungal infections in persons with poor oral hygiene or in those who suffer from systemic illnesses such as leukemias (blood cancer) diabetes, renal failure, anaemia, deficiency state and AIDS/HIV diseases. A common form of stomatitis develops in ill-nourished children and in adults during fevers, who have infected gums and septic teeth and those with badly fitting dentures. People who do not maintain proper oral hygiene especially during serious ailments, their lips, tongue and gums are effected which become inflammed, swollen and painful. Tongue is furred and there is foul smell.

In addition in bacterial and fungal diseases, various types of viral infections also produce vesicular type of stomatitis. Here there are small vesicles surrounded by redness. These vesicles generally rupture, leaving behind grey ulcers. These are extremely painful present on the inner surface of the lips, cheeks and margins of the tongue. The person generally a child or a young adult has features of toxaemia like fever, malaise, etc.

Deficiency diseases like anaemia, pellagra, and beri beri often produce a tongue which is red, swollen and inflammed. Person suffers from a burning sensation in the mouth which is increased by hot and spicy food.

A number of people suffer from single or multiple painful superficial ulcers which occur on the mucus surfaces of the mouth, tongue and buccal mucosa. These ulcers are small and have erythematous border. The exact cause of these ulcers is not known except that sometimes they are present in deficiency states and gastrointestinal disorders.

Management of stomatitis includes care of the mouth hygiene. Tongue should be kept clean. Teeth be cleaned carefully and antiseptic gargles and mouth wash be used two to three times a day.

To prevent irritation and soreness of the mouth, soothing ointment containing glycerine (gelora) be applied locally on the mucosa.

For secondary bacterial infection appropriate antibiotics have to be given.

General nutrition of the person has to be taken care of and deficiency state, if present, has to be corrected. If stomatitis is due to systemic diseases (blood disorders, malignancy, heavy metal poisoning, skin disorders, metabolic disease, uraemia), bacterial, fungal and viral infections, appropriate treatment has to be instituted under the guidance of a physician.

Glossitis

It is inflammation of the tongue accompanied by soreness and redness. A number of causes may be responsible for this and these range from excessive abuse of alcohol, spices, smoking, tobacco chewing, vitamin B complex deficiency, anaemia to metabolic disorders like diabetes mellitus. Use of dental prostheses, ill fitting dentures, inflammed gums or ill spaced teeth are other factors responsible. These cause excessive salivation and tingling sensation in the tongue.

Anorexia (Loss of Appetite)

It is a very common problem which effects almost every person at some or other time. Anorexia means loss of appetite and lack of desire to eat. It is a symptom complex of number of conditions which may be mild in nature while in some it may indicate a serious ailment.

Anorexia mainly occurs in gastrointestinal disorders but may also occur in other conditions.

Emotional disturbances top the list of causes responsible for it. Anxiety, depression and any condition producing stress, the first casualty is lack of desire to eat. In case of liver disorders, loss of appetite and aversion to food is one of the earliest symptom. Surprisingly, cases of hepatitis take their breakfast with relish and as day passes their desire to eat just goes away.

List of causes producing loss of appetite is lengthy one and ranges from acute infections, congestive heart failure, renal failure, gastritis, pulmonary tuberculosis, malignancy anywhere in the body, myxoedema, chronic alcoholism to drug toxicity.

As said, loss of appetite is a symptom of some underlying disease which must be investigated and treated accordingly. Nature just draws attention to the problem by this symptom.

Nausea and Vomiting

Nausea and vomiting are almost interrelated and anybody suffering from it presents the same picture. Any person who complains of a feeling of nausea has a discomfort like sensation and there is a desire to vomit which constitutes the act of bringing out the stomach contents. Severe form of vomiting is accompanied by retching.

Nausea and vomiting are a symptom complex of number of diseases ranging from gastrointestinal disorders (acute/chronic gastritis, food poisoning, gastroenteritis, carcinoma stomach, intestinal obstruction, viral hepatitis, cirrhosis of liver, acute/chronic cholecystitis, acute/chronic pancreatitis), systemic causes (renal colic, diabetic acidosis, food poisoning, chronic alcoholism), Neurological disorders (Migraine, brain tumour, vertigo, encephalitis, meningitis) to drug toxicity (digitalis, morphine, anti-tubercular drugs, chloroquine, metronidazole). Nausea/vomiting is of common occurrence in the first trimester of pregnancy. Similarly, any unpleasant site or smell may produce either nausea or vomiting.

Anybody presenting with either of the two conditions should be properly examined, investigated and treated accordingly.

Abdominal Pain

Pain in abdomen is a very frequent problem and many people suffer from it. It may be mild, moderate or severe in nature which may require urgent management.

It may be superficial or deep and is mainly of two types. One which arises from structures constituting the abdominal wall while the other variety arises from abdominal viscera due to their distension, spasm, obstruction or ischaemia. Occasionally pain may be referred to abdomen from disease elsewhere and classic example of this is pain in a case of heart attack which may be referred to upper part of abdomen. Similarly in diseases of the thorax and spine pain may be referred to abdomen.

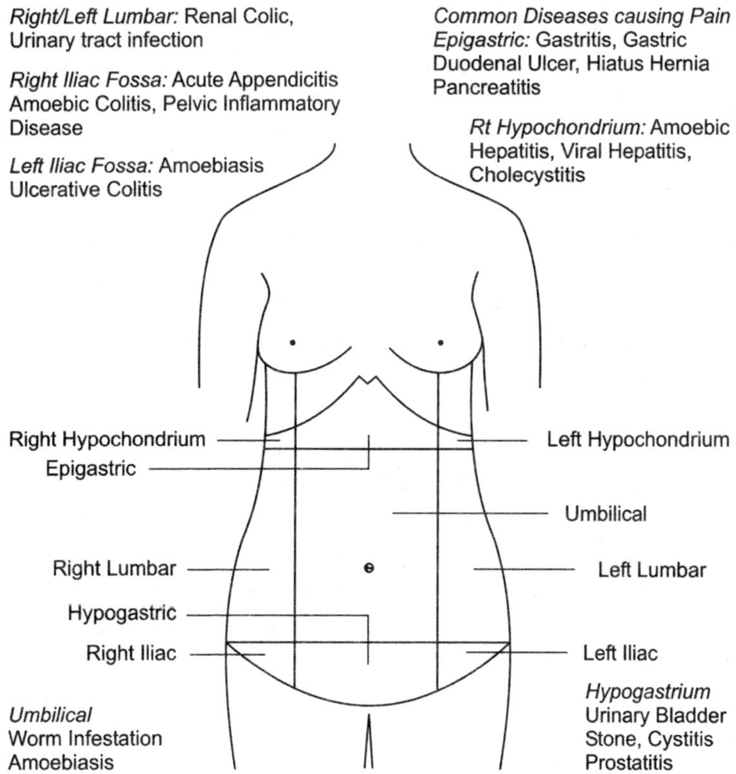

Nine regions of Abdomen

In every case of pain abdomen, the basic approach is to the site of pain, character, severity, radiation and referral to any site along with accompanying symptoms and how relieved.

In cases of gastric or duodenal ulcer, there is tenderness in the upper part of abdomen while in acute cholecystitis there is tenderness to right of costal margin with catch in breath. Pain lower down on right side is present in a case of acute appendicitis. Similarly, cases of renal colic have pain in lumbar region radiating down to inguinal region.

Cases of amoebiasis have a diffuse sort of pain in abdomen.

Presence of an acute pain of recent origin points towards a more serious ailment while chronic pain in abdomen is due to inflammatory conditions. Pain in renal, ureteric stone or gall stones is colicky in nature, generally of short duration and is relieved after the acute attack passes away and patient may have symptom-free period afterwards. A chronic pain lasting for weeks accompanied with weight loss and poor health points to the possibility of malignancy.

Radiation of pain is equally important. Pain of gall bladder disease is referred to shoulder or angle of scapula: pancreatitis pain to back and renal pain to the groin. Some cases of gastric or duodenal ulcer have relationship with food. While pain in gastric ulcer is increased after intake of food, the pain of duodenal ulcer is relieved after taking food. A fatty food may trigger an attack of acute cholecystitis.

In addition to pain, other symptoms like vomiting (appendicitis, cholecystitis, pancreatitis) dysuria and blood in urine (renal colic) when present will help in making a diagnosis.

As compared to men, women suffer from pain in the abdomen of varying intensity during menstruation. Inflammation of pelvic structures in females is also an important cause of pain in abdomen. It may be acute or chronic.

Acute pelvic inflammatory disease (PID) is a common problem affecting women in their reproductive period. Early recognition and effective treatment of the condition is important in preventing complications. It is an infective inflammation of the upper genital tract caused by organisms ascending from vagina and then infecting tubes. Women who have the highest risk of developing the disease are generally menstruating. It is a polymicrobial infection and number of organism, ranging from N. gonorrhoeae, monilial, trichomonas, aerobic and anaerobic organising are responsible. Pain in lower abdomen is by far the most frequent symptom. Pain is usually diffuse, dull and present on both sides of the abdomen. Pelvic inflammatory disease (PID) is the most common diagnosis in a young woman complaining of pain in lower abdomen.

So a person who comes complaining of pain in abdomen shall require a number of investigations. Rise of blood count will indicate inflammatory conditions of abdomen. Urine should be looked for albumin and pus cells. A battery of biochemical tests, radiological studies, ultrasound of abdomen and endoscopy are other procedures indicated. But the choice of investigations shall depend on the advice of the treating physician who shall carry out the relevant investigations after making a thorough examination and reach the relevant diagnosis.

Only a brief resume of various probable causes of pain in abdomen has been enumerated and final advice is to be given by the treating doctor.

Worm Infestation

A very common problem especially in young children and adults is the problem of worms which are present in the intestines and act as parasite who derives not only food but also blood from their victims producing a strain on the person's vitality. People who suffer from worm infestations are poor specimens of health suffering from constant pain in abdomen, loose bowels, general weakness and lack of vitality. There are number of worms like hook worm, thread worm, round worm, tape worm, etc. which infect man. Most of the people harbour more than two or three types of worms because the same factors which predispose a person to suffer from one also predisposes him/her to get the other worm infestation. How the worms behave in the body in their course of either entry or development has also its own effects. Thus round worms migrating from place to place in the body may not only block the intestines by their sheer physical

Worm	Name	Zoological Name	Disease
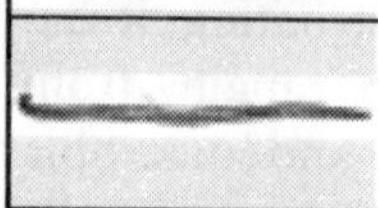	Roundworm	Ascaris Lumbricoids	Ascariaris
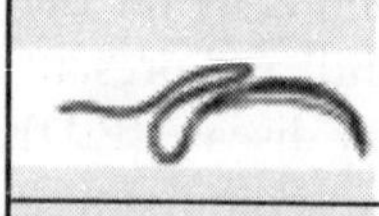	Whipworm	Trichuris Trichiura	Trichuriasis
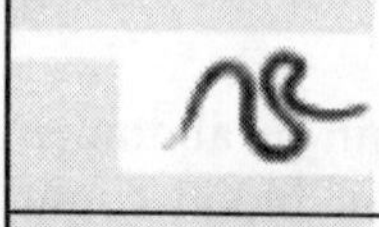	Threadworm	Stronglyoides stercoralis	Stronglyoidasis
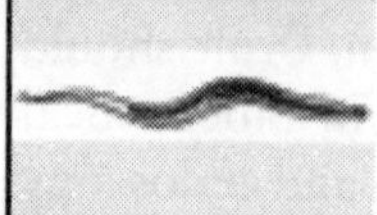	Pinworm	Enterobius vermicularis	Enterobiasis
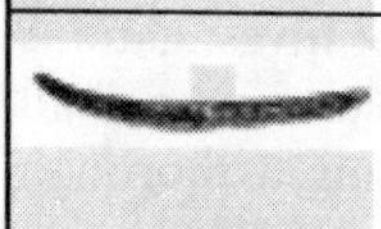	Hookworm	Ancylostoma duodenale & Nectar Americans	Ancylostomiasis
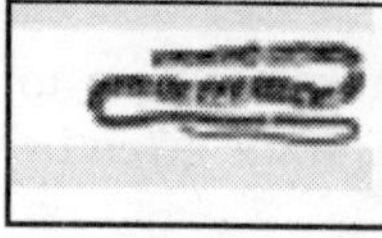	Tapeworm	Taenia saginata	Taeniasis

Common worms which infest humans

number but may perforate the intestinal wall or even rupture one of the important organs in the body like liver.

Similarly, hook worm larvae enter into the body through exposed skin and start a form of reaction accompanied by itching. When hookworm gets lodged in the intestines, it sucks blood constantly and produces iron deficiency anaemia. Pin worms are thread like worms which commonly involve children and constantly produce irritation round about anus.

Tape worms pose an acute danger to man as they are likely to invade vital tissues and cause serious damage. Tape worm infection is acquired by eating either raw or uncooked meat which contains larvae of these worms. There are mainly two types of worms—Beef tapeworm (Taenia saginata) and Pork tapeworm (Taenia Solium). Infection occurs when either infected beef or pork meat is eaten.

SYMPTOMATOLOGY OF COMMON WORMS

Types of worm	Symptoms
Pinworm (Enterobiasis)	Itching round anus. Lack of sleep. Restlessness, fatigue, irritability, prone to bacterial and other infections.
Roundworm (Ascariasis)	Intestinal colic. Loss of appetite and weight. Dry cough. Breathlessness, acute intestinal obstruction, rupture of liver, blockage of bile duct.
Threadworm (Strongyloidiasis)	Pain in epigastric region, diarrhoea, nausea, vomiting, allergic reaction, itching.
Hookworm (Ancylostomiasis)	Itching and burning at place of entry. Epigastric burning, sallow skin, anaemia, alternating diarrhoea and constipation, general weakness.
Whipworm (Trichuriasis)	Loss of appetite, and weight. Nausea, vomiting, diarrhoea, anaemia, abdominal discomfort.
Tapeworm (Taeniasis)	Hunger, pains, abdominal discomfort, flatulence, neurological symptoms.
Fish (Broad) Tapeworm	Increased appetite, abdominal discomfort, weight loss, diarrhoea, anaemia, Vitamin B_{12} deficiency.
Dwarf Tape-worm (H. Nana)	Diarrhoea, abdominal discomfort.

Dog tapeworm inhabits the intestines of dogs, jackals or wolves but not of man. Man becomes infected from it in peculiar ways, i.e., by drinking unclean water and eating raw vegetables contaminated with animal faeces. Close contact with dogs in the form of handling and fondling also produces infection. This tapeworm produces the condition called hydatid disease.

Besides these, there are fish tapeworm, Dwarf tapeworm (H. Nana), whipworm (Trichuriasis) etc. which produce number of symptoms ranging from vague abdominal discomfort, increased appetite, nausea, vomiting, etc. Once a person is diagnosed to be suffering from worm infestation, treatment must be taken under medical supervision. At the same time it is important to take adequate steps to eradicate the disease.

It is important to have proper sanitary facilities. Human waste should not be used as fertilizer in field so that propagation of worms does not take place. Do not go bare footed in the field.

One should avoid eating raw vegetables and fruits which have not been washed properly. Avoid infected or undercooked meat. General hygienic measures all round should be followed. Hands must be washed thoroughly after using the toilet. Nails of hand be trimmed regularly and let not any dirt accumulate under them.

It is quite common that worm infestation is present in other members of the family as well. So to completely eradicate them, all other family members be also dewormed at the same time and all members must adopt meticulous hygienic measures.